THE
PARISIAN DIET

Editor: Kate Mascaro
Translated from the French by Anne McDowall
Text adaptation: Margit Feury Ragland
Recipe adaptation: Helen Woodhall
Design and Typesetting: Gravemaker+Scott
Proofreading: Nicole Foster
Indexing: Cambridge Publishing Management Ltd
Cover illustration: Kanako Kuno
Printed by Worzalla in Wisconsin, United States
© Flammarion, S.A., Paris, 2013

13 14 15   3 2 1

Hardcover ISBN: 978-2-08-020139-3
eBook ISBN: 978-2-08-129557-5

Dépôt légal: 01/2013

DR. JEAN-MICHEL COHEN
FRANCE'S FOREMOST NUTRITION EXPERT

THE PARISIAN DIET

*How to Reach Your Right Weight
and Stay There*

Flammarion

CONTENTS

FOREWORD

ONE AFTERNOON IN JUNE 2007, I entered the waiting room of Dr. Jean-Michel Cohen's medical practice in Paris. It was two o'clock in the afternoon and the room was crowded. I sat down next to a heavy-set older woman. Chatting with her, I learned that she had arrived in Paris that morning from Bordeaux, a five-hour journey. Her consultation was scheduled for three o'clock. She was early, but couldn't afford to be late because there was a three-month waiting list for appointments. Mine own meeting was scheduled for two thirty. In a few minutes, I was going to meet the most famous French nutritionist. The one who appeared on television several times a week, the favored doctor of overweight celebrities: singers, actresses, politicians, etc. Even though I was a bit nervous, I was really looking forward to meeting him.

It was the day after the official launch of the first iPhone by Steve Jobs, which marked a major revolution in mobile phone history. I was particularly struck by two things that Jobs had said: "Apple is going to reinvent the telephone" and it would put "your life in your pocket." These two catch phrases may have seemed far-fetched or pretentious at the time, but we take them for granted today. In 2002, I had created Anxa.com—an online start-up based on a simple and ambitious idea: to revolutionize health and fitness by using new technologies (internet, mobile, and desktop). My technique was largely inspired by Jeff Bezos's philosophy for developing Amazon.com. I had the privilege of speaking with Bezos in 1999, during the Amazon France launch where he advised me that the key to success in the twenty-first century would be the quality of the customer service. His work both persuaded and inspired me. And so I placed the individual at the center of our business strategy by developing a particularly proactive level of customer service. To do so, my team maintains daily contact with each client, individually, in order to check on their progress and satisfaction, and to offer encouragement. Anxa.com had already established a reputation in Paris by 2007, and the company was poised to revolutionize the online health, nutrition, and fitness market.

In just a few more minutes I was going to ask Dr. Cohen if he would partner with us. The conversation I'd had with the woman from Bordeaux had convinced me of the potential merits such a collaboration. I knew that with someone of Dr. Cohen's caliber on our team, we would be in a position to help hundreds of thousands of people all over France. And it would no longer be necessary for them to put up with a three-month waiting list, or to spend ten hours traveling travel back and forth to Paris. I imagined online coaching not as a replacement, but as a useful accompaniment to the components that already existed: the initial consultation to make a diagnosis and to get off to a good start, the indispensable monthly appointment for tracking the patient's progress, the diet books for informing patients in detail on what steps they needed to follow to succeed in their weight-loss efforts.

Dieting can be hard. There are so many mixed messages and so much temptation everywhere. The first step has to be your own commitment, and then you need a plan that will keep you motivated over time. To succeed, you need to make a promise to stay with the program. That is what I said to Dr. Cohen at our first meeting and what initially got him on board; his own work with his patients was based on the same concept. And that was the beginning of our collaboration in the Anxa.com online coaching service, which has helped five hundred thousand people in France lose weight over the past five years.

So it's with great pride that I accepted Dr. Cohen's request to write the foreword to his first "American" book. He knows that, just like him, I love the United States—I lived in Dublin, Ohio for a year during high school where I got my first taste of what it was like to live the American dream—and that, just like him, I will not feel a true sense of professional success until the day I make a difference there. Which is why, to supplement this book—and drawing from the lessons of Jeff Bezos and Steve Jobs—I have developed theparisiandiet.com, an online coaching site that offers personalized daily emails, videos, and discussion groups, as well as *The Parisian Diet* Smartphone application.

It is true that in France, we enjoy a certain quality of life, we have a vision of happiness, and pursue our famous *joie de vivre*. These are three wonderful characteristics that we like to share with the world. Our lunches can famously last up to two hours. Even when they are less extravagant, they remain an important part of our day and are often shared with friends and colleagues. Dinner, which can take at least as long as lunch, is always devoted to our families. France also has a long history of cuisine, gastronomy, nutrition. So I am very proud, as a devoted fan of the United States, to introduce you to *the* diet solution from Dr. Cohen, the man who, for so many years, has helped millions of French people to lose weight and stay in shape. In this book you will discover his best advice and practical tips for shedding your excess pounds and starting a new life.

This time, it's the right time; now it's up to you to lose weight by improving the way you eat and starting your new Parisian-style life, "*la vie en rose.*"

— Fabrice A. Boutain

PREFACE

T HE FACT THAT I BECAME A NUTRITIONIST was no accident. I waged
my own battle with weight loss.

My mother, after several challenging events in her life, began gaining weight and, over time, became obese. It was the 1970s and diet gurus
were all the rage. I saw her go from one quack to the next, each one promising the moon yet always leaving her to gain back even more weight.

Like mothers everywhere, she adored her oldest son, yours truly.
She manifested her love by feeding me, probably more than I needed. I
became a chubby kid, then obese. As a result, I was bullied at school. In
the locker room, I felt humiliated by the stares that my flab attracted.
I was uncomfortable interacting with others, especially with girls. In a
nutshell, my weight was linked to everything that made me unhappy.
But I was totally incapable of following a diet—I couldn't even fathom
trying. And I certainly couldn't count on my mother, who kept reassuring me of all of my other positive qualities.

The first time I set my mind to losing weight was after a young
romance went sour. I hated my body and decided that it was the cause
of the break-up. I threw myself into a severe, self-imposed diet. I ate a
slice of bread with butter in the morning and had meat and a piece of
fruit every day for lunch and again for dinner.

During the diet, I exercised intensely, which took my mind off my
broken heart. I lost weight quickly. With each pound that melted away,

I became increasingly motivated to lose the next one. That said, following the period of rapid weight loss, I developed a kind of food phobia, in which everything seemed to be forbidden. My mother, of course, was extremely worried; she discouraged my weight-loss efforts and constantly pressured me to eat.

Later, when I began my medical studies, I didn't realize that my desire to help people stemmed from a desire to help my mother and myself. The day I met the talented man who ran the hospital nutrition center was the day I found my future career. I dove into the world of nutrition with a passion that still drives me today, and I was fortunate to become one of the early pioneers of this science. Back then, when I arrived at the hospital to treat patients, the other doctors often thought I was a chef!

After thirty years of treating patients in France—where I also hosted a popular reality television weight-loss program—I have shifted my focus to the growing problem of obesity in America.

I've admired the United States for a long time now, and have held a strong emotional connection to the country since my childhood, when, living in war-torn Algeria, the American soldiers stationed there were a symbol of security and hope for my family and me. I remember occasional interactions with soldiers who treated me with kindness and entertained us by sprinkling their effervescent powder onto the ground (it was standard-issue powdered drink mix, but it—and they—seemed magical to my young eyes). My family eventually fled to France to escape the horrors happening in our homeland. There, I fell in love with American culture, in particular with Hollywood's sensational heroes—from Superman, to Batman, to Rocky. So today, I am perplexed to see a country that has always exuded such strength and vitality now allowing the world to view its typical citizen as obese and its national cuisine as junk food. How is it possible that Americans—always cutting edge and renowned for succeeding at every endeavor—still haven't found a solution to their national obesity problem?

I feel compelled to help. Virtually all of the discoveries in the field of nutrition that I studied in medical school came from doctors and researchers in the United States, who were my precursors and role models. Today, the country's best scientists struggle to resolve the greatest epidemic facing their health industry. I see so many Americans struggling with their weight, in increasing numbers, and professionally, I want to make a difference.

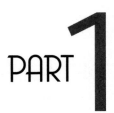

PART 1

BATTLING THE BULGE

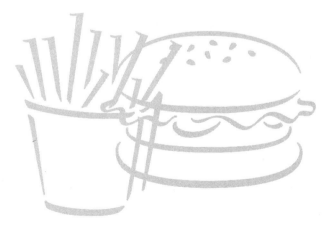

INTRODUCTION

EVERY YEAR COUNTLESS FAD DIETS EMERGE with miracle promises, yet none provide a lasting solution for managing your weight. For those who have tried and failed repeatedly, this is a painful reality. Once you step into the world of dieting, you are unlikely to ever get out again. The desire to shed pounds quickly becomes an obsession: you wake up thinking about how to lose weight and go to bed dreaming of being slim by morning. It's time for a realistic diet, based on a healthy balance of eating enough so you're not hungry yet reducing your calorie intake so you slim down—all while relishing each meal.

With the Parisian Diet, I'll teach you how to change the way you eat, but not radically, so that you'll be able to stick with it. I'll show you how to break old habits and clear up misconceptions about food, such as the belief that the only way to lose weight is through abstinence. You can't maintain an important life change if it is based on deprivation; that's a sure-fire recipe for failure! I offer a sustainable solution. It's not another flash-in-the-pan diet that will suck you into a cycle of yo-yo weight fluctuations. It's a new approach to eating, drawing from a European tradition of regularly spaced meals and featuring delicious, healthy, and easy-to-prepare recipes that will bring a taste of France to your table.

Just because you're on a diet doesn't mean that fun is off the agenda. I will give you clear strategies for eating out, show you how to celebrate special occasions without ruining your diet efforts, and help you deal with cravings when they hit. Use my list of alternative ingredients (see pages 76–79) in recipes to substitute anything you don't like to eat.

With this diet, education is the key. You will only succeed in losing weight permanently when you learn to do so intelligently. I explain how to recognize the food industry's tactics that get us to eat more and teach you how to put into context the unrealistic ideal of beauty prevalent in the media. I encourage you to seek deep within yourself to uncover the real cause for your weight gain, and share strategies that will help you become—and stay—slim. My straightforward plan includes practical dieting checklists and pointers on how to avoid common food traps. This book blows the whistle on false claims in the food industry and in fad diets in order to help you learn to diet better.

For several years, I have been analyzing American eating patterns, looking at the whole food chain and the habits that impact the way Americans eat. In the Parisian Diet, I address the physical, psychological, and cultural factors that impact our complex relationship with food. The solution I offer is a French one, born from my understanding of the problem from both a scientific and personal perspective. This customized weight-loss program, with personalized coaching also available online at www.theparisiandiet.com, will permit you to steadily lose six to eleven pounds per month. And in the end you'll see that it's not just about losing weight. It's about accepting your body and its contours and transforming it into everything you want it to be.

French Lessons

The Parisian Diet is modeled on healthy French eating habits, which offer substantial health benefits and protective features. Implementing French traditions alone can improve your health dramatically. Consider this: On average French people spend around two hours per day eating meals. The French consume more than 90 percent of their daily calorie intake at mealtimes. Conversely, Americans consume less than 80 percent of their calories at breakfast, lunch, and dinner. That means more than 20 percent of Americans' calories come from snacking between meals—a substantial amount. A recent study by Kiyah Duffey and Barry Popkin of the University of North Carolina at Chapel Hill shows that, over the past thirty years, American adults have increased their number of daily meals and snacks from three and a half to five, which amounts to an increase of 400 calories per day. The study concludes that "efforts to prevent obesity among U.S. adults (and among adults in other developed countries) should focus on reducing the number of meals and snacks people consume during the day as a way to reduce the energy imbalance caused by recent increases in energy intake."[1]

In France, mealtimes are considered a real and necessary ritual, even when they don't last for very long. In contrast, in the United States, eating often is seen more as a mechanical act of "refueling"; something that can be done at the same time as other activities. Sixty-eight percent of French people eat lunch at home during the work week. This number is far lower in the United States, where "about 65 percent of employees eat lunch at their desk or don't take any lunch break at all."[2] And the number of American families dining together, especially during the week, has been plummeting. In the past, family time revolved around the dining table. Our modern lifestyle, backed by the development of new food technologies—snacking, sandwiches on the go—ensures that opportunities to get together to eat are becoming increasingly rare. Whereas mealtimes and food once brought groups of people together, today they isolate them. We eat from vending machines and drive-thru windows. We move ever farther from the ways of our ancestors. In the United States there have been some strides to offset this negative shift, but the results may be even worse. We're being sold—with the help of advertising and branding—new,

100-percent artificial food products that are supposed to recreate this sense of community in the form of "family-sized" boxes of macaroni and cheese, frozen pizza, and more.

Americans, as a result of these factors, are now the most obese people in the industrialized world.[3] The numbers are not pretty. In France, the proportion of obese people with a Body Mass Index of 30 or greater is relatively low compared to other developed countries at 16.9 percent of the population, compared to 33.9 percent of Americans.[4] I have spent a great deal of time studying why this is the case. Most of it has to do with these cultural and behavorial differences: First, the French are actively interested in cooking and cuisine. Pleasure is deliberately emphasized as a fundamental aspect of the eating experience and the quality of the ingredients is very important. A perfect hors d'oeuvre is appreciated for its flavor, color, texture, and presentation—and each morsel is savored. Americans, on the other hand, attach more importance to the nutritional content of food and to the quantity, with the assumption that more is better. For the French it is the *joie de vivre* and the "naturalness" of foods that guarantee good health. The French do not eat simply to nourish themselves; eating is an activity in and of itself that begins with writing the shopping list and continues as we prepare a meal and sit down at the table to enjoy it with our family. This is a key difference between the French and Americans. Eating together at regular times is a priority in the Parisian's daily routine. It helps us to avoid snacking throughout the day, which is critical in the fight against excess weight and obesity.

1   Kiyah J. Duffey and Barry M. Popkin, "Energy Density, Portion Size, and Eating Occasions: Contributions to Increased Energy Intake in the United States, 1977–2006," *PLoS Medecine*, vol. 8, no. 6 (2011), e1001050.doi:10.1371≠journal.pmed.1001050. From www.plosmedicine.org (accessed October 1, 2012).
2   From Eve Tahmincioglu, "America's Lunch Hour on the Endangered List," published on http://lifeinc.today.com/_news/2012/01/18/10175875-americas-lunch-hour-on-the-endangered-list?lite (accessed August 23, 2012) with findings based on a Right Management™ web survey, 2011. © 2012 NBCNews.com
3   World Health Organization (WHO), "Global Database on Body Mass Index: Maps," apps.who.int/bmi/index.jsp (accessed July 22, 2011) as cited in "U.S. and Global Obesity Levels: The Fat Chart" on http://obesity.procon.org (accessed August 23, 2012).
4   Ibid.

PARISIAN TIPS FOR YOUR DAILY ROUTINE

1 **Enjoy your meal and indulge yourself from time to time.** This
is the most important element in succesful dieting. If you force
yourself to eliminate all of your favorite foods, you'll eventually give
up on the diet. Instead, if you slip up or simply can't resist a craving,
take the time to enjoy your occasional splurge. Just be sure to make up
for it with a recovery plan meal (see page 268), and then resume
your diet.

2 **Space meals out regularly** throughout the day and rediscover
the pleasure of sharing a meal instead of leaving each member
of the family to nibble away on whatever they can find in the fridge
and the cupboards at every hour of the day and night. This will help
to limit snacking between meals with the added bonus of promoting
good relationships within the family.

3 **Take a break.** Three times a day, take time off to eat—a minimum
of twenty minutes per meal—and pay attention to what you eat. Don't
distract yourself with anything else. Reading, watching television,
working on the computer, or engaging in other activities while you eat
are particularly hazardous because they focus your attention elsewhere,
which prevents you from tuning into the clues that your body sends
to acknowledge when you're full. It's very easy to keep on eating as
if you're on autopilot until all of the food is gone, unless you give
your meal your undivided attention.

4 **Focus on making each meal a pleasure.** Now that you're focused
on your meal—get all of the senses involved. Savor each mouthful.
Really taste every bite. It may sound funny, but when you take
a moment to look at and smell your food before tasting it, it can
enhance the overall experience, making you more fully appreciate
and feel more satisfied with your meal.

5 **Get back into the kitchen.** Return to home cooking with simple recipes
and fresh ingredients, rather than prepackaged, ready-made meals,
which contain excessive amounts of salt, saturated fats, and trans fats,
and which make it difficult to achieve a balanced diet.

6   **Reduce portion sizes**. When you overload your plate and then feel compelled to eat everything on it, you often end up eating more than you really need—and continue eating even after you feel full.

7   **Drink water** throughout the day.

CHAPTER 1

STRIVING TO BE THIN: AGAINST ALL ODDS

ONE SIZE FITS ALL: AN IMPOSSIBLE IDEAL

W E ARE AT ODDS WITH OURSELVES. At the dawn of the third millennium, fat is out, yet the majority of us are just that. While we're more obsessed with body shape than ever before, few of us are happy when we look at ourselves in a mirror. We are much like the evil queen in Snow White: when she sees her reflected image and learns she is no longer fairest of them all, she becomes enraged and depressed. Who hasn't felt this way? Our well-being is dependent upon the way we view ourselves, no matter who we are and where we live in the world.

From Paris to Hollywood, and in every small town in between, the belief in inner beauty has been largely abandoned. Instead, week after week, we monitor the changes in the waistlines of our favorite celebrities. Who has put on or lost the most weight? We barely discuss their current performances, as their talents of singing or acting have taken a backseat to how they look. We scrutinize their derriere or their legs, in the hope that these celebrities, when they lose weight, will divulge the magic formula. And some of them do lend their name to endorse a wonder product—even though they might not have tried it themselves—and we follow them blindly, credit card in hand. In our minds we create a personal ideal of beauty that is insidiously oppressive and destructive. And this is done with the complicity of the press, the fashion world, the media, and even doctors!

Who hasn't heard both of these statements from their doctor: "You must lose weight; your health depends on it" or "Don't diet like that; it's dangerous for your health"? How can you sort through these mixed messages?

The current situation is not unique to the United States. It's happening everywhere. Since the media have such a firm grasp on defining our ideal of beauty—and news organizations have become increasingly international—distinctive regional, national, and continental notions of beauty are becoming blurred in favor of identikit characterizations of one size fits all. The same supermodels grace the covers of magazines everywhere; the same actresses are shown in New York, London, and Hong Kong; the same idols appear on the small screen and in video clips. A homogenous world style has emerged. And when those idols are matchstick thin, androgynous, anorexic, or flaunt silicon-enhanced breasts, an unhealthy so-called norm emerges that millions of women attempt to emulate.

And this "accepted standard" is far from reality. "Since the mid 1970s, the proportion of people who are obese ... has increased sharply in many countries."[5] Take my country, France, for instance. More than 49 percent of the population has a Body Mass Index of 25 or greater, qualifying them as either overweight or obese.[6] The numbers in the United States are even worse. A staggering 66.9 percent of Americans today qualify either as overweight or obese.[7] It's a global problem, but one that is particularly acute in the United States where "the proportion has doubled since 1980, and a third of all [American] adults—more than seventy-two million people—are now classified as obese."[8]

THE EVOLUTION OF EATING

Society is constantly evolving, often in a positive direction. Clearly, our eating habits have changed over the generations. Traditionally, eating was limited to three meals a day, plus a few small snacks. But today, forget about mealtimes; we sweep aside the rules, satisfy immediate desires, and lose all sense of discipline. It's chaotic behavior. Nothing is structured anymore, it's all about impulses and temptations. Over the past three decades, eating between meals has increased significantly. "The prevalence of snackers increased from 71 percent in 1977 to 97 percent in 2003–2006," and "the percentage of energy intake from snacking ... increased to 24 percent."[9] What luxury! But at what price?

Globalization is one reason for the changes in eating patterns. In the past, some cultures enjoyed a hearty morning meal while in others the evening meal was most substantial. Today, we swap ideas and traditions: croissants and pain au chocolat are popular in England; twenty-four-hour bakeries with items that blend all cultures are popping up across the United States; brunch menus in France are gaining popularity as quickly as pancakes can be served; and Italians are starting their day with scrambled eggs. We are all enriching one another, but all of these different eating habits can be overwhelming and lead to a destabilization in our lifestyle as well as our bodies. We are being seduced without considering the consequences as we eat whatever, whenever. Even a product as simple as the potato is not immune. It comes mashed, baked, as hashbrowns or tater tots, ready to fry, chopped, sliced, in soups and salads—and eaten with all sorts of sauces and toppings.

The consequence of this explosion of flavors and their easy availability is that we multiply opportunities to eat faster and without exerting effort in preparation. It also encourages guilt-free eating with the explosion of "diet" options intended to promote weight loss, yet which ironically have become a factor in weight gain. So we end up living in a world where physical slimness is placed on a pedestal, while at the same time we are bombarded with enticements to buy and consume fat-laden food. This is particularly sadistic for overweight people who are simultaneously stigmatized and encouraged to buy products that lead to weight gain.

The Magnetism of Advertising

Who's to blame? Is it the media? Advertising? Perhaps. I am sometimes startled by ads, especially those that make out processed or otherwise unhealthy food to be something that it's not.

Two classic French television ads illustrate my point.

The first one preys on nostalgia and our desire to rekindle the family connection at mealtimes. A young man is eating a slice of toast with jam. We see him remembering the time when, as a child, he enjoyed his grandmother's homemade jam. He breaks into a smile. The consumption of sugar-laden jam is used to evoke an image not only of the past but also of the close relationship he shared with his grandparents. Such wistful flashbacks feed viewers with the desire to eat this purely industrial jam.

The other commercial shows a party on a beach; a group of cool young people with sculpted bodies dancing, kissing, having fun. There is an overall sense of happiness and freedom. One of the youngsters throws a bottle in the air and the top comes off. All of them are drinking the same soda and having a great time. Through the magic lens of advertising, the drink has been infused with the connotation of youth, freshness, and joy. Why do we choose to buy it: to quench our thirst or to be like them?

I'm sure you've seen commercials like this no matter where you live. With constant new product inventions, we are bombarded at every turn—on TV, in magazines, on billboards, and especially at the grocery store. They all have one aim: to instill a desire in consumers to buy, eat and drink, and open their wallets. This is especially troubling for someone who wants to lose weight. We are faced with hundreds, if not thousands, of products that lead us to believe they are healthy and therefore "on our side" when, in reality, their claims are intent on increasing our consumption and therefore their producer's profits. Labels in every aisle boast their diet-friendly benefits: "Low-calorie," "No Sugar," "Low Fat," High in Fiber," "Fat Burning," "Meal Replacement," and the list goes on and on. Under such conditions, how can we resist the temptation to succumb to all these promises, or even worse, to give up entirely and grab a box of cookies?

STOCKING UP AT THE SUPERMARKET

At the grocery store, a multitude of products line the shelves, each promising they won't put inches on your waist while they somehow simultaneously will improve your health. While strolling the supermarket aisles, you stumble across a yogurt drink you saw advertised on TV that morning. The supermarket manager saw the ad, too, and displayed the product prominently. Your brain has now been influenced, twice, so your hand automatically reaches for it and puts it in your cart—without even a glance at the label. In addition, the family pack is great value, so you buy two giant containers of a sale item, with no thought to its health benefits or lack thereof. Similar scenarios play out throughout the store.

The same supermarkets that propose healthy or diet products also offer the richest and most mouth-watering food choices. That's why, lost in all these media messages, obsessed by the ideal of beauty, each of us tries to find a more-or-less satisfactory solution, a shaky compromise between the good and not good, the healthy and unhealthy, and we end up taking all the pleasure out of eating. Just as bad, we've forgotten how to plan meals by choosing food that is fresh, truly delicious, and simply good for us.

While your intention may be to pick up the ingredients for a healthy family dinner, it's not surprising if, because you're pressed for time, you grab something that is quick and processed yet boasts some type of health benefit, and head to the register. You get home with more food than you needed. In the following days, not wanting to let anything go to waste, you end up eating everything you bought.

If this sounds only too familiar, don't lose hope. I'm here to help.

- **Deciphering Food Labels: Portion Size**

In addition to the lure of advertising, packaging on the products in the supermarkets touts their desirable nutritional properties, but what is really in the food you're buying? How many calories are you actually consuming? We can't spend our time dissecting every product we plan to consume, armed with a little calculator. However, we should be vigilant, to ensure that we eat the portion size that we intend to and so we know what is in the food we buy.

The concept of "per portion" confuses us more than anything else. Although it provides us with a standardized gauge of nutritional and energy values, in a fairly consistent manner throughout the food industry, manufacturers are nevertheless free to define the portion size for their product as they see fit. Recently I picked up a candy apple at a grocery store. When I turned the product over to look at the label, I noticed that a serving was only 126 calories. That seemed quite acceptable, and eating it was an enticing proposition. However, upon reading the label more closely, I realized that the portion was not the whole apple, but only half of it! Can you imagine me politely eating half of the apple and leaving the other half in the fridge once it was unwrapped? The manufacturer had fooled me into feeling reassured about the calories per portion, but it was the actual portion size that in no way corresponded to what I was about to eat.

This happens constantly as I make my way through a supermarket. A box of my favorite cereal contains 110 calories per serving, but the serving is just three-quarters of a cup. A little experiment reveals I typically pour out close to two cups, which adds up to a whopping 293 calories. A small bag of chips proudly sports the label: "No Trans Fat and Only 100 Calories." Sounds good to me. Until I see that it's 100 calories per one-ounce serving. That's a mere handful, not the whole bag.

- **Don't Make Assumptions**

One popular product, the granola bar, has become particularly significant, because many of us eat them as part of the diets we follow or as a snack to satiate hunger during the afternoon. Unfortunately, most of us are victims of the widespread misconception that all granola bars are healthy. For instance, when I did a quick comparison of one randomly chosen granola bar and a Snickers bar, I discovered that the granola bar contains 471 calories and the Snickers 475. Not much of a difference there. Another bar contains more fat than two Oreo cookies.

In eating granola bars, we hope to tame our hunger pangs, but in fact, the sugar they contain (sometimes as much as you'd find in a serving of chocolate ice cream), may calm our cravings for a short while, but will increase our desire to eat an hour later. Without us noticing, they simply awaken our appetite. So before grabbing your next granola bar, which is very easy considering its practical packaging, consider a piece of fruit instead—which comes in its own handy and all-natural packaging!

- **What's Inside?**

Finally, for a bit of fun, I've included one of the food labels that most amused me:

Wheat Flour, Water, Shredded Low-Moisture Part-Skim Mozzarella Cheese (Part-Skim Milk, Cheese Culture, Salt, Enzymes), Shredded Reduced Fat Reduced Sodium Mozzarella Cheese (Pasteurized Part-Skim Milk, Nonfat Milk, Modified Food Starch, Cheese Cultures, Salt, Potassium Chloride*, Natural Flavors*, Annatto [Color], Vitamin A Palmitate, Enzymes [*not found in Regular Mozzarella Cheese]), Cooked Seasoned Pizza Topping (Pork, Water, Mechanically Separated Chicken, Textured Vegetable Protein [Soy Protein Concentrate, Caramel Color], Spices, Salt, Sugar, Sodium Phosphate, Paprika, Pork Flavor [Modified Corn Starch, Pork Fat, Natural Flavors, Pork Stock, Gelatin, Autolyzed Yeast Extract, Sodium Phosphate, Thiamine Hydrochloride, Fatty Acids, Propyl Gallate], Caramel Color, Spice Extractives, BHA, BHT, Citric Acid, Cooked in Pork Fat or Beef Fat or Vegetable Oil), Tomato Paste, Pepperoni (Pork, Beef Salt, Spices, Dextrose, Lactic Acid Starter Culture, Oleoresin of Paprika, Flavoring, Sodium Ascorbate, Natural Smoke Flavor, Sodium Nitrite, BHA, BHT, Citric Acid), Partially Hydrogenated Soybean Oil, Sugar, Red Bell Peppers, Green Bell Peppers, Contains Less Than 2% of Soybean Oil, Wheat Gluten, Black Olives, Onions, Bleached Wheat Flour, Salt, Yeast, Potassium Chloride, Modified Food Starch, Sodium Bicarbonate, Sodium Stearoyl Lactylate, Sodium Aluminum Phosphate, Dried Parsley, Spices, Dried Garlic, L-Glutamic Acid, Citric Acid, Ascorbic Acid (Flavor), Beta Carotene (Color). (8% Sausage & Pepperoni.)

It's hard to believe that we're talking about a pizza!

While it's not an everyday occurrence, often when I'm in Paris and want to please my children, I buy some pizza dough, cover it with some tomato paste, sometimes add ham, and top it all with mozzarella. Doesn't that sound good? It just goes to show that cooking at home can be quick and simple, and it's the best guarantee that you know what you're putting in your mouth.

5   Kiyah J. Duffey and Barry M. Popkin, "Energy Density, Portion Size, and Eating Occasions: Contributions to Increased Energy Intake in the United States, 1977–2006," PLoS Medecine, vol. 8, no. 6 (2011), e1001050. From www.plosmedicine.org (accessed August 23, 2012).
6   World Health Organization (WHO), "Global Database on Body Mass Index: Tables," apps.who.int/bmi/index.jsp (accessed July 22, 2011) as cited in "U.S. and Global Obesity Levels: The Fat Chart" on http://obesity.procon.org (accessed August 23, 2012).
7   Ibid.
8   Duffey and Popkin.
9   Carmen Piernas and Barry M. Popkin, "Snacking Increased among U.S. Adults between 1977 and 2006," The Journal of Nutrition (American Society for Nutrition, 2010), pp. 326, 327.

CHAPTER 2

WHY IT'S SO HARD TO LOSE WEIGHT

AN ALL TOO FAMILIAR STORY

SUZANNE'S STORY IS A COMMON ONE, and one with which you're likely to identify. Suzanne was thirty years old when she first went on a diet, restricting what she ate. She lost her target of eleven pounds on her own within a couple of months. Unfortunately, six months later, she had gained it all back. That's when she went to a drug store to buy some (not inexpensive) plant-based gel capsules to help her lose weight. She tried them, but they had little effect.

One of her friends suggested she try a mail-order weight-loss program that came complete with creams, gel capsules, and an array of brochures. Suzanne was easily persuaded and started the program right away. She lost seven pounds this time, but still had four that wouldn't budge. She noticed that she was snacking more often between meals. To appease her cravings, she started buying granola bars after seeing ads in magazines and on television about their benefits. She also filled her refrigerator with low-calorie foods and healthy snacks, began eating bran cereal with a teaspoon of wheat germ for breakfast because she'd heard it was good for diets, and always carried a big bottle of mineral water around with her.

But when she weighed herself she was dismayed. Not only had she failed to lose the four pounds she was hoping to lose, but she had put on another nine, which meant that she now had a total of thirteen pounds to lose rather than the original eleven.

Upset but determined, she went to a personal trainer, who, as luck would have it, had just bought a "revolutionary" new machine. In ten sessions (at one hundred dollars per visit) she would lose her excess pounds without even trying.

She also bought a book written by a doctor who explained that to lose weight she needed to eliminate sugar from her diet, but that she could consume as much fat as she liked. It was worth a try. After all, her friend's colleague had lost twenty-two pounds on the diet.

Suzanne conscientiously followed the advice in the book, consumed not a single ounce of sugar, and went twice a week to the trainer, who hooked her up to his machine. "It worked!" the trainer said. Suzanne lost one and a half inches from her waistline and more than one inch from each thigh. She was happy. But her bathroom scale gave her less favorable news. She had lost only four and a half pounds. Furthermore, when she took her waist and thigh measurements at home, she didn't get the same results as her trainer. Perhaps she put the tape measure in the wrong place, she thought.

But how was she going to lose those remaining nine pounds? She decided to change her method and tried a new diet featured in her favorite celebrity magazine. But with so many complicated recipes it was impossible to stick to it.

She was thoroughly fed up, so Suzanne went back to see her pharmacist, who assured her that protein powder would do the trick. To lose weight quickly, all she had to do was drink a protein shake for lunch. She decided to try it. For three weeks it was "adieu lunch, bonjour shake." She drank four liters of water a day, snacked only on granola bars, ate frozen diet meals for dinner and—miracle!—lost all the weight. She felt happy, proud, and good about herself.

Six months later, she had gained back all the weight, plus another seven pounds. Her original goal was slipping further away and she was really upset. Something must be wrong with her. But who should she go to about her problem? It was time to turn to modern medicine. Her family physician sent her for a battery of blood tests. Everything was fine. He prescribed her a mild sedative, to calm her anxiety. It wasn't cheap, but it helped her sleep. It didn't, however, help her lose weight. Frustrated, she turned to snacks to cheer herself up.

Then she heard about a specialist who had helped a lot of people lose weight using his own patented capsules. The attentive receptionist and the sumptuous interior of the consulting room were reassuring, although the nonrefundable fees made her break into a cold sweat. There was no doubt about it, the physician told her, she suffered from a problem of sugar regulation, associated with poor absorption of nutrients into her blood stream. He handed her a preprinted "prescription," that she needed to get filled at a specific pharmacy. At the drug store, the pharmacist handed over the medication, not covered by insurance, for three hundred dollars.

A week later, Suzanne was no longer sleeping, felt the need to urinate constantly, and was arguing with everyone. She went back to her family physician, who reviewed the prescription and told her that it could have killed her. He advised her to make an appointment at a hospital specializing in weight loss, which she did. But it took three months to get an appointment.

Finally at her consultation, they took more blood tests and told her to return in a month. Thirty days later, she found herself waiting in a large room with ten other patients. After a group pep talk, she met with a nutritionist, who questioned her about her eating habits and sent her back to the waiting room. Two hours later, the nutritionist presented her with a diet plan. Happy at last to have found a scientific solution, Suzanne read the plan:

- *Breakfast: bread, yogurt, fruit.*
- *Lunch: raw vegetables, broiled meat with more vegetables, fruit.*
- *Dinner: soup, fish, yogurt, fruit.*

No kidding.

Disillusioned, she returned home, folded the paper in four, put it in a drawer, and cried.

Months later, another expert told her that surgery was her only option. She agreed. When she spoke to her husband about it, he got angry. He told her that her five-year obsession had become ludicrous.

She always failed, but he loved her just they way she was, and besides, at her age, it was normal to be a bit plump.

She was speechless. She didn't go under the knife, but instead went to see another physician. When she failed at this diet, too, she became truly depressed. Her weight kept increasing until she simply gave up.

Two years later, Suzanne walked into my consulting room. She just couldn't shake her desire to lose weight. She had fallen into the yo-yo dieting trap too long ago.

"Suzanne, why do you want to lose weight?," I asked her.

"To feel better about myself," she replied.

"But why else?"

She no longer knew. Her quest to lose weight was so old that she had forgotten how it started. It had become an obsession that she could no longer control; it had invaded every aspect of her life and made her unhappy. Less than ten years after her initial attempt to lose eleven pounds, she was now thirty-three pounds heavier. She no longer knew how to eat, and could no longer gauge when she was hungry or when she was full. Sometimes she ate a lot, at other times nothing at all. Furthermore, she often felt tired, had trouble sleeping, was self-conscious around other women, had lost her libido, and had stopped wearing makeup or paying attention to how she dressed. She felt miserable. And she had spent thousands of dollars. Unfortunately, the yo-yo dieting trap often causes you to lose more from your bank account than from your hips.

How do so many people fall into the yo-yo dieting trap? Where does this desire to lose weight at any price come from, which spurs people to try any method possible, from the most rational to the most miraculous? What leads so many women, in particular, to deprive themselves for years for such unconvincing results?

It goes something like this: On Monday morning, Suzanne arrives at work and has coffee with her friends and colleagues. They talk about the weekend, sharing what they'd done, where they'd been, movies they'd seen, and meals they'd eaten. And then someone complains that she has to lose the pounds she put on over the holidays.

It begins to take root in conversations with friends. A friend's worry about her weight alerts Suzanne to her own extra pounds and the thought surreptitiously creeps into her head. "Hey, maybe I should drop three or four, or even five or six pounds, too."

Around noon, her meeting convenes for a lunch break and the whole committee goes to a restaurant together. The daily special is a burger with French fries. Or, there is inevitably one healthy choice on the menu. Uh-oh! Here comes another opportunity for contamination. Suzanne sees her colleagues divide into two groups: the healthy eaters and those who can't resist the burger. Which should she choose? That will depend on what those seated closest to her choose; she usually follows along with whatever the group does.

At five o'clock, Suzanne goes home. On the way she stops at the supermarket to pick up a few things. She makes her way down the aisles, chooses her food, carefully reading the product labels. Nonfat or low cal, enriched with something, without something else, diet option, healthy option, and the list goes on. Once again, uh-oh! Her mind is like a sponge: it's trying to absorb all this "information" that insinuates that she, too, should monitor what she's eating and tighten her belt a notch or two. Traps in the supermarket are everywhere as food displays reinforce the notion of weight control and slimming down.

These minor incidents accumulate throughout her day, and Suzanne becomes increasingly anxious about her weight.

At home, she turns on the television while she prepares dinner. A few video clips precede a popular dance program. Here we go again!

None of the young dancing girls, with their skin-tight jeans, high heels, and narrow hips, has the slightest physical imperfection. Suzanne is now grappling with the dangers of an inattainable fantasy. With these television stars as her point of reference, she begins to day-dream—which spirals into self-criticism: she's too plump here, a bit too big there. In short, she doesn't fit the "norm" displayed on television.

Her meal finished, the mental torture continues with the parade of reality TV stars. On screen is a woman who will gain fame and money simply because she is "beautiful." So Suzanne compares herself to this woman, whose figure in no ways resembles her own. In between episodes, she sees conflicting ads—those for weight-loss programs followed by those for snacks that are reportedly healthy. When she gets into bed, she flips through her favorite magazines with the headlines, "Lose Weight with this Diet," "How To Get Rid of Your Saddlebags," and "Lose Ten Pounds in Two Weeks." The fashion pages show trends that she could never pull off because they would high-light her figure's imperfections. She turns off the light with these thoughts running through her head. The same scenario repeats itself all week long.

The problem, once the habit of yo-yo dieting has firmly taken root in Suzanne's mind, is that the initial reasons for wanting to lose weight (just a little bit so her body would be better proportioned) will fade and die, replaced by a raging battle. Her fight against excess inches will consume her and she gradually will forget her original motives for losing weight. In her quest for new solutions she will lose her grasp on reality. She will become a diet addict without realizing it.

Extreme Weight-Loss Methods

It's striking how many people who want to lose weight have used a dangerous or grueling weight-loss method at least once. We abhor such practices and the pain they cause, yet every time we hear about someone who loses a significant amount of weight through such a scheme, we get excited, ignoring the most basic precautions. The prospect of losing weight dramatically, even if it means resorting to risky or outlandish methods, continues to entice.

Over the last few years, there have been no shortage of "new" weight-loss methods. The sum total of one doctor's advice to his patients is to eat nothing but an apple a day. Another uses acupuncture, which, he claims, will dispel hunger pangs. A third uses laser beam technology on the zones of the body that are allegedly responsible for obesity. These various "wonder treatments" follow in a long tradition of similar scams. The ingredients for promoting weight-loss methods remain unchanged: a little publicity, a little medicine, and a few spectacular testimonials. The quantity and order in which those ingredients appear varies according to the product, but the main objective is always to sell the greatest number at the highest price and as fast as possible.

I will concede that these extreme methods, including diet pills and weight-loss surgery, sometimes work—at least for the time being. A person who has lost weight dramatically will usually maintain their slimmed-down weight for a while. But once he or she gets accustomed to the result, the pleasure of eating will replace that of being slim. This is how the mechanism of yo-yo dieting operates. And once we start the cycle, we may as well accept the idea of a variable weight with periods alternating between being overweight and "normal." We might even find logic in the repetition of these swings. After all, two steps forward and one step back still add up to a step forward. However, unsettling research from the United States has shown that mortality rates among obese people whose weight had fluctuated a lot was much higher than for those whose weight had remained stable.

The more times you yo-yo, losing and regaining weight, the harder it becomes to lose weight the next time. Suzanne certainly experienced this. It happens because of two antagonistic hormones in our body: leptin and ghrelin. The job of the first is to cause satiety (the sensation of being full); the second, to increase appetite. Yet the more a person loses weight then gains it back, the more the level of ghrelin will gradually increase and the level of leptin decrease. What a terrible injustice that when we most need to lose weight, hormones stop us from doing so and, moreover, increase our appetite! To make matters worse, sleep deprivation, which is very common in adults, increases the secretion of ghrelin and decreases that of leptin. The fatter we are, the more we risk gaining weight once we multiply our attempts to lose weight ... unless we change our behaviors once and for all.

Causes of Weight Gain

Having treated some thirty thousand patients over the years in my medical practice, I have encountered myriad reasons why people gain weight. A diverse range of psychological and behavioral reasons are commonly associated with excess weight (incidentally, these same causes can have the opposite effect and trigger eating disorders causing malnutrition, as well). I often see patients who use weight gain as a form of protection; the body changes itself to serve as a shield against the outside world.

Two factors combine to bring on weight gain: a decrease in the expenditure of energy and/or an increase in energy intake (calories). This can be triggered by an increase in food consumption or a change in eating habits, but there are also many other factors—such as medication, menopause, quitting smoking, stopping exercise, and lifestyle changes—that can also be to blame.

• Medication

Weight gain is a common side effect of certain medications. When this happens, those taking the drug must pay special attention to their diet, decreasing the number of calories they take in, or increase physical activity. With your physician, you should discuss the effects your prescription drugs have on weight and devise solutions for keeping your weight in check.

• Menopause

During menopause, it's common for women to gain ten to fifteen pounds as the body increases its capacity to store food and reduces its rate of expending energy. At this time of her life, a woman is often faced with a number of unsettling changes: she may feel the early effects of aging or struggle with "empty nest" syndrome when her children leave home. The anabolic effect of hormone replacement therapy may also have an impact on weight. In addition, the decrease of certain hormone levels, particularly reproductive ones, leads to a drop in cell activity, further decreasing energy expenditure. Balancing diet and exercise is again the key.

- **Exercise and Physical Activity Level**

If you stop playing a sport that you once practiced regularly or otherwise decrease the amount of exercise you're getting, the reduction in energy expenditure often leads to weight gain—unless, of course, food intake is controlled.

- **Quitting Smoking**

When someone quits smoking, the problem is twofold. Nicotine triggers energy expenditure, so stopping smoking can lead to a weight gain of around nine pounds because the body is burning fewer calories. If weight gain exceeds that figure, it means that the smoking habit has been replaced by eating to compensate. To help patients lose weight, or simply maintain the same weight when they quit smoking, a physician must address the patient's anxiety and diet. Nicotine patches are also effective.

- **Life Changes**

Changes to your daily routine can provoke weight gain. And sometimes the link between the weight and the external change is surprising. For instance, it is not uncommon to see some patients gain weight after relocating. The repercussions of moving are both psychological (you need to get your bearings) and material (your routine is different). As a result, an increase in appetite compensates for the unsettling effect of such an upheaval. Your diet may also be affected by where you move. For example, if you live on the West Coast of the United States, you could find your diet completely disrupted if you move to the East Coast or to another region, where the variety and availability of foods differ significantly from what you're accustomed to. Even a time or climate change can have an effect on your eating habits and regular mealtimes.

I Can Relate: Case Studies

Below are the compelling stories of some of my patients, which I hope will help people faced with similar struggles. When the problems that beset a person remain unresolved, he or she can gain weight; when such worries are addressed, sustainable weight loss becomes possible. Awareness of the underlying reason is key in being able to address the behavioral patterns that lead to chronic weight gain and you may benefit from professional support in tackling these factors as you begin your weight-loss plan.

- **Daily Temptations**

John, who is fifty, is a salesman for a large corporation. He usually has a light breakfast before leaving the house. When he gets to work, he makes himself a cup of coffee. Morning breakfast meetings often include pastries. He usually restrains himself for the first fifteen minutes, but then caves in and indulges. At lunchtime, very busy, he eats at his desk while he continues to work. Even if he wants to order a healthy dish, his favorite—a bacon, turkey, and mayo sandwich—often calls his name. When he gets home in the evening, he doesn't eat right away. To relax, he pours himself a drink, accompanied by some peanuts or potato chips.

In the morning, John's wife Sylvia prepares breakfast for the children. She serves breakfast cereal, fruit juice, toast, and cheese, based on healthy eating guidelines she picked up at the grocery store that she wants her children to follow. Preparing breakfast makes her hungry and she often nibbles on the children's leftovers. She runs errands all morning and returns at noon to grab a quick bite. Most of the time she makes do with a chunk of cheese and a granola bar or a cookie from the cookie jar. When the children get home from school, she prepares their snack ... which presents a new temptation for her to eat. If she gives in, she'll feel guilty and frustrated. Even when she refrains, she can't resist a few of the bits and pieces they left uneaten. In the evening, the children are hungry before John gets home, which means that Sylvia ends up cooking twice every evening: two more chances for temptation. When her husband gets home, she joins him for a cocktail—more calories to deal with.

Every so often, both John and Sylvia decide to diet. John goes to work on an empty stomach. At the office he sees his colleagues eating muffins or bagels with their coffee; he turns to his work. The morning doesn't go very well. By midday, he's thinking about his lunch meeting, hoping that the caterer will have something good. While everyone else chooses whatever they want from the buffet, he picks food that fits in with his diet. He finishes his lunch in a pretty bad mood and gets back to work. His frustration grows all afternoon, and by four o'clock, he has a major sugar craving. He could go and get himself a candy bar from the vending machine, but knows he'll just feel guilty afterwards, so he refrains. By the time he gets home, he's in a foul mood. His frustration grows with each passing day. Soon, he begins cheating on his diet. Because he has trouble finding a balance between his difficulty in losing weight and the daily temptations he faces, John's best option is to find time to exercise a few times a week.

For Sylvia, the problem with dieting is even more acute. Instead of being at work with only the vending machine to satisfy her desires, she's at home, faced with cupboards stocked with temptations. Is it any surprise that within a week or two, both John and Sylvia give up on their diets?

- **Microstresses**

Mary, a young woman in her thirties, came in for a consultation at the end of September, because she had been struggling to lose a few extra pounds for several months. For years she had been accustomed to fluctuating between two weights: she weighed four and a half pounds more in the winter than in summer, but would quickly restore the balance in the spring by following a low-calorie diet. This year, as usual, she started her usual routine but to her delight, she lost nine pounds in May and June. And during her summer vacation, she had eaten whatever she wanted without resisting. When she returned home, she was pleasantly surprised to discover that she had lost another couple of pounds. However, at the end of September, she noticed that although she hadn't changed the quantity of food she normally ate, and consumed less than what she'd had during her vacation in August, she had gained eleven pounds. She was therefore convinced that she was getting fatter even though she was eating less. She felt like her body was changing and that she was doomed to continue gaining weight.

But there's nothing miraculous about weight gain or weight loss. Mary's mistake was that her perception of the "quantity" she was eating did not address the fact that the food choices she was making in September were more calorie-dense than what she had chosen during her diet and on vacation.

An experiment along these lines was undertaken in Denmark a few years ago. Over the course of eight days, some twenty volunteers agreed to be filmed inside an apartment. During the week, video cameras carefully recorded everything that these human guinea pigs put in their mouths, from the moment they woke up until they went to sleep. At the end of the experiment, the organizers asked the volunteers what they had eaten during the week. To their great surprise, there was a 30 percent difference between the food they remembered eating and what they had actually consumed.

In fact, none of us is capable of saying exactly what we ate during a day, from morning to evening, when questioned about it a week later. If we are asked what we ate on a given day, we will recall the most memorable dish—a sirloin steak or a salmon fillet—but not the rest. Munching on a sandwich, grabbing a piece of candy from a colleague's desk, or finishing off a meal with some chocolate are all harmless enough, and are often unconscious actions, but they all have a caloric value.

The real issue for Mary lay in accurately taking stock of what she was eating. What were her eating habits before vacation? Getting to the truth depended on her answer. I questioned her about her diet since returning from vacation. She had followed it carefully, eating in the morning, at noon, and in the evening. And if, she felt hungry in the afternoon, she would munch on an apple or allow herself a cup of nonfat yogurt. Nothing that would justify such a spike in weight gain.

When I questioned her more in depth, I also learned that she was experiencing some difficulties at work. One of her colleagues was being very aggressive and stirring up trouble for her with her superiors. Sometimes, without Mary understanding why, the colleague would stop speaking to her. In fact, this colleague was depriving Mary of the pleasure she usually drew from her work, and created what we call a microstress. In addition to the headache at work, which she said she could handle, Mary wanted to move but didn't have the down payment for her dream apartment closer to the office. In short, another microstress. Mary also had car trouble; she needed to get major repairs done and was worried about how she would be able to foot the bill.

Mary's life is fairly typical: she faces everyday concerns that don't seem major in and of themselves, but the accumulation of these aggravations had become a major cause of anxiety. So much so that rather than enjoying a sunny day and chatting with a friend, Mary woke up thinking about her car, fumed about her colleague on her way to work, and pined after the apartment on her way home at the end of the day. As she was increasingly less content with her life, she offset her frustrations by finding solace in food.

When Mary was on vacation, free in body and mind, she ate only when she was hungry rather than at rushed mealtimes during a hectic work day. Away from home, her only preoccupation was choosing what to do with her free time. Without the temptation of food in easy reach, as it was at the office, she spent time outside from dawn to dusk, with no snacking fodder in sight.

But when she returned to reality, stress caused her to wolf down her meals and snack on chocolate mid-afternoon. And at mealtimes, while she thought she was eating less than when on vacation, she was choosing richer foods and eating larger portions of them. Her stresses led her to increase the amount of food consumed, and, with an unbalanced diet, she inevitably gained weight, which became a new stress factor to add to the others.

Mary's story illustrates one of the most pervasive phenomena of contemporary life: microstress, or the accumulation of microstresses, which creates significant frustrations. Without someone who can listen to and understand us, the easy answer to counter these attacks is likely to be food. Dieting in this context has a chance of success only if the problems are brought to light. If you remove outside stresses, and are able to take things in stride again, your food intake will no longer be impulsive and will stabilize. If you are not chronically overweight, you will return to your normal weight.

- **Family Dynamics**

Christelle, age thirty, was afflicted with a considerable weight problem: she was 5 feet 7 inches tall and weighed 286 pounds. She was constantly dieting, but each ended in dismal failure as she regained as much weight as she had lost. Nevertheless she was persuaded that, with perseverance, she would eventually find a solution. Beneath her apparent detachment, however, I sensed a certain tension, an agitation. Her movements were jerky, and she spoke quickly. She displayed a deceptively casual air, but she often ran her hand through her hair—a host of signs that betrayed an inner emotional turmoil. Her anxiety was visible, but she wouldn't acknowledge it, even though she felt comfortable with me. Her problem, she told me, was that she was eating balanced meals, but would occasionally binge. Or, she went on to explain, when she started to eat a particular food—often potato chips, chocolate, or pasta—she wouldn't be able to stop.

I prescribed her a standard restrictive diet of around 1,400 calories a day along with an antidepressant to be taken after lunch. I explained to her that the particular type I was giving her helps combat impulsive behavior, which is the truth, but I also knew that this antidepressant would help her overcome her anxiety. She was an intelligent woman, successful in her career as a sales director for a large pharmaceutical company, and despite an initial reticence, she conceded.

Our consultations continued over the course of several weeks and Christelle quickly lost weight: in four months she dropped from 286 to 216 pounds—a magnificent result. I had reason to be pleased with the progress and was looking forward to seeing the follow-up, when a strange phenomenon occurred. She lost another twelve pounds in two weeks, but during the third week, she gained half of it back again. She told me that the antidepressants had changed her life, but I could see that she was particularly sad that week, a bit lost, and her thoughts were elsewhere.

One day, when she arrived at my office very irritable and uptight, I asked her what was going on. "Nothing," she answered me brusquely, in a way that intrigued me further. I weighed her: she had put on four and a half pounds. As I was cautioning her that she shouldn't continue to yo-yo like this, she burst into tears and told me that she had just spent a dreadful weekend with her family. And there, I uncovered the mystery: she had a sister, married with two children, while she herself was single, and every two or three weeks, the whole family got together at her parents' house in Brittany. That weekend, her nephews had been particularly rowdy, and Christelle criticized her sister for not disciplining the boys. She expressed anger at the disrespectful way the boys treated their grandparents, and her outburst created a scene. Her parents replied that the boys' behavior didn't bother them and reprimanded Christelle's interference; her sister told her to mind her own business and to take a look at herself before judging others. In short, Christelle felt doubly stung.

Christelle finally broke down and shared with me the dynamics at work in her family. Christelle had for a long time been her parents' favorite. While Christelle was single, her sister was visibly jealous of Christelle's superior professional success, a situation she balanced out by focusing her energy on her husband and children. Christelle's weight loss was a new source of jealousy that, in short, was challenging the balance of family dynamics.

In order to rise above the situation, Christelle decided to temporarily suspend contact with her family. The break saddened her, but she thought it was necessary. Her decision was a good one. Christelle has dramatically lost weight, started dating, and is working on rebuilding her family relationships.

• A Controlling Influence

Sandra, twenty-five years old, 198 pounds, and 5 feet 5 inches tall, had the usual story: she wasn't eating and yet was putting on weight. At every consultation, I noticed that she hadn't lost an ounce, and yet she assured me that she was following her diet to the letter. The next time I saw her, I suggested that she keep a food diary to itemize everything she ate. She returned the following week, with the notebook meticulously filled out, but with no change in her weight. The only difference this time, was that her mother had accompanied her and was sitting in the waiting room. And her mother was very eager to speak with me.

With Sandra's consent, I invited her mother Martha into my office, where she explained to me that her daughter was very immature and was constantly eating between meals, stuffing herself with chocolate and other candy. During this diatribe, Sandra didn't open her mouth.

I noticed her exasperation but she remained silent. The mother began attending our weekly meeting, and I grew increasingly irritated by her. Martha was so invasive that Sandra was manifesting her rejection via her body, by symbolically swallowing her anxiety in the form of food. Sandra was conflicted because she felt guilty for being a burden to her mother, who had been abandoned by Sandra's father, and so she never wanted to upset her mother. Martha's primary occupation was taking care of her daughter, and as a result, she was completely smothering her. When I met with Sandra's fiancé, he explained to me that her mother was always at their place, telephoned several times a day, and would turn up unexpectedly. In fact, Martha was trying to live her daughter's life by proxy, an intrusion against which Sandra was trying to protect herself by increasing in size. And ever since Martha became involved in her efforts to lose weight, Sandra no longer wanted to slim down. A parent who is too involved in his or her adult child's life is an extremely common problem. Children in this situation often have serious difficulty coping and many turn to food in order to escape.

- **Marital Troubles**

Carrie, who worked in a bank, came to see me to lose forty-four pounds. A rather dowdy woman, she sported a haircut thirty years out of date, wore thick glasses, was conspicuously unkempt. She looked as if she were in her fifties, but in fact she was only thirty-eight. When I questioned her about why she wanted to lose weight, she stated it was for her health.

Carrie lost weight very quickly and her appearance gradually began to change. She also began to open up more. She didn't dwell on her two children: they were doing well at school and both had a good relationship with her. The snag, I guessed, was with her husband: she adored him but they had not been intimate for two or three years, without her knowing why. Her husband explained that he just didn't enjoy intimacy anymore. He even suggested, to her shock and dismay, that she take a lover. Carrie couldn't imagine sex without love, and she in turn suggested that her husband see a doctor, advice that did not go over well.

Because her partner refused to seek help and she had trouble acknowledging that he shared responsibility for the situation, she assumed the blame and in turn made herself physically undesirable.

Rather than expressing dissatisfaction with her love life, she chose, unconsciously, to change her body.

At the same time, she struggled to resign herself to this new image, and now that she began to shed the excess pounds, Carrie literally began to blossom week after week. As she got back into shape, she began to enjoy taking care of her appearance again. Her husband didn't know what to think of her sudden transformation. And then, one day, she arrived looking fully content. When I asked her the reason for her happiness, she said with a wide smile that she had reconnected with her husband again.

Certain forms of depression commonly result in the sufferer losing interest in themselves, and weight gain is one of the first manifestations of this. In cases of severe depression, when nothing holds any interest, a person will reject the notion that his or her body could be an object of desire.

- **Sign of Health**

Sixty-year-old Yvonne came to see me because she wanted to lose about twenty pounds, an excess she had been carrying for the past year. She had been diagnosed with breast cancer, but had been clear for one and a half years. Without realizing it, she herself had diagnosed a problem. During treatment for cancer, patients lose weight. Following the end of treatment, and for about a year afterward, almost without exception, they gain it back. After that, many say that they want to lose weight, but often can't manage to do so. In fact, subconsciously, we associate cancer with being thin, and so in the mind of ex-cancer sufferers, being large means that they are healthy again. It can take a woman, torn between the fear of being skinny and the desire to be "like other people," about a year to become convinced that she is well again. Slimness then changes status in her mind and comes to represent a renewed recognition of her body, a sign of her confidence in her wellness and in the future.

- **Adjusting to Retirement**

Edward, sixty years old, had trouble breathing and arrived in my office wheezing. He told me the story of his weight gain, in which alcohol had played a significant role. His life was filled with professional lunches and pleasurable moments dining at home. This businessman, who was nearing the end of his career, was elected mayor of his town. A few years later, he sold his company but then suffered a crushing political defeat. He suddenly found himself doubly retired and without his many professional responsibilities, Edward was not only bored, but had also lost his self-esteem. He was feeling an inner emptiness that he was filling in two ways: first by treating himself to his favorite foods, and then by going overboard and eating to excess. This man whose life had been so full was now literally stuffing his body.

This form of weight gain is extremely common. Upon retirement, many people use food to fill the void in their life. The cause is not only due to the sudden lack of occupation but also the loss of self-esteem that comes from having lost one's bearings, and the accompanying fear that the end of one's working life may also presage social death. The role of the doctor, in such a situation, is to show that it's possible to be retired and still have an active role to play in society, via friends, family, and even volunteer work. When retired people take an interest in others, study a new subject, or become active in organizations, they noticeably combat depression.

How to Avoid the Yo-Yo Diet Trap

1 **Take a step back.** Let's face it: we have quite a knack for looking at situations through a magnifying glass! Don't allow your mind and emotions to be overwhelmed by your environment. Snap things back into perspective and get a clear focus on the world around you. Being able to laugh about things often does wonders for diffusing negative thoughts.

2 **Get rid of preconceived ideas.** Think critically and, above all, with careful reflection. An ad that promotes a flawless standard of beauty is unrealistic. Remember that software is used to retouch the smallest imperfection. Don't forget that marketing gurus are looking to seduce you and they are very talented in that arena.

3 **Work on yourself.** If you feel the need to be listened to or counseled, don't be ashamed, just admit it and go for it. A therapy session, far more so than fruitless inactivity, will enable you to gain a clear perspective.

4 **Be realistic.** It's great to set a goal and work towards it, but nothing is more discouraging than striving for a goal that you'll never be able to reach. Take stock of what's really important to you and, with an objective eye, establish an "inventory" and a plan of action that is within your grasp.

5 **Trust yourself.** There is no reason why you can't reach a realistic goal. Write down a list of your motivations and reread them regularly. This will enable you to stay focused on them and will help you move forward at times of doubt.

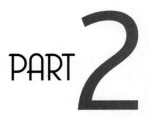

PART 2

THE PARISIAN DIET

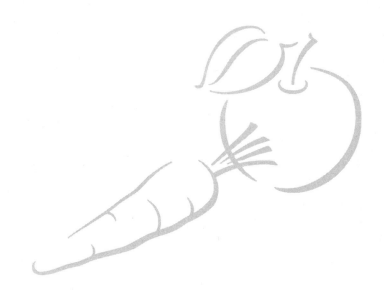

CHAPTER 3

CALCULATE YOUR RIGHT WEIGHT: SET YOUR GOAL

I HOPE THAT IN READING THIS BOOK, you've come to realize that the idea of magically morphing overnight into an airbrushed super-model on the cover of a magazine is not how you're going to gain control of your weight and your figure. But just what *is* your goal? You need to set your "Right Weight." The Right Weight is the weight you should be able to attain without the fear of piling on excess pounds when you resume a normal diet or eating routine. This is vitally important because you want to avoid regaining at all cost. Every time you lose and gain back weight your body produces new cells that have the ability to store even more fat than before. That's why most people who lose weight on quick and easy diets end up weighing more in the long run.

So how do you figure out what is the Right Weight for you? I've developed a formula, which will help you identify your genetically stable weight. This is the weight that you can reach, will be happy with, and the one that you will have the best chance of maintaining over time.

THE RIGHT WEIGHT FORMULA

A   How much did you weigh when you were 18 years old, without dieting (e.g., 150 lb.)?

B   How much did you weigh at your heaviest, excluding pregnancy weight (e.g., 210 lb.)?

C   How much did you weigh at your lightest after age 18, with or without having dieted (e.g., 140 lb.)?

D   What is your current weight (e.g., 200 lb.)?

Add together your answers to questions A and B and divide by 2 (e.g., 150 + 210 / 2 = 180 lb.). This is figure Y.

Add together your answers to questions C and D and divide by 2 (e.g., 140 + 200 / 2 = 170 lb.). This is figure Z.

Add figures Y and Z and divide by 2 (e.g., 180 + 170 / 2 = 175 lb.). **This is your Right Weight**.

So now that you have it—a number in black and white that represents your potential stable weight—you may be surprised to find that it is higher or lower than you expected. But keep in mind that this is an achievable goal for you. It's a starting point based on what your body at this moment in time can reasonably achieve. The length of time it will take to reach that goal depends on the difference between your current weight and your goal weight, but you will see that this three-phase diet plan will offer you the flexibility to stay with your weight-loss program until you reach your Right Weight. By then, you will have formed the good habits you need to maintain this weight over the long term. You should continue to monitor your weight and can implement the Café phase or the Bistro phase (see pages 85–107 and 109–163) for two to three days to keep yourself in check if you notice a slight weight increase of five pounds. Once you have maintained your Right Weight for a period of six months to a year, you should also check your Body Mass Index to see if your current weight is in the normal range. If not, you should use the Right Weight formula again, using your new stable weight as the "D" variable, therefore setting a new Right Weight goal. You can continue progressing over time until you achieve a BMI that is neither overweight nor underweight by implementing the diet and achieving your Right Weight. Just remember that before recalculating your goal, you need to have maintained your Right Weight for at least six months straight.

BODY MASS INDEX TABLE

BMI	16	17	18	19	20	21	22	23	24	25	26	27	28	29	30	31	32
Height (feet/ inches)	Underweight			Normal						Overweight						Body We	
4'10"	77	82	87	91	96	100	105	110	115	119	124	129	134	138	143	148	153
4'11"	80	85	90	94	99	104	109	114	119	124	128	133	138	143	148	153	158
5'0"	82	88	93	97	102	107	112	118	123	128	133	138	143	148	153	158	163
5'1"	85	90	96	100	106	111	116	122	127	132	137	143	148	153	158	164	169
5'2"	88	93	99	104	109	115	120	126	131	136	142	147	153	158	164	169	175
5'3"	91	96	102	107	113	118	124	130	135	141	146	152	158	163	169	175	180
5'4"	94	100	105	110	116	122	128	134	140	145	151	157	163	169	174	180	186
5'5"	97	103	109	114	120	126	132	138	144	150	156	162	168	174	180	186	192
5'6"	100	106	112	118	124	130	136	142	148	155	161	167	173	179	186	192	198
5'7"	103	109	115	121	127	134	140	146	153	159	166	172	178	185	191	198	204
5'8"	106	112	119	125	131	138	144	151	158	164	171	177	184	190	197	203	210
5'9"	109	116	122	128	135	142	149	155	162	169	176	182	189	196	203	209	216
5'10"	112	119	126	132	139	146	153	160	167	174	181	188	195	202	209	216	222
5'11"	115	122	130	136	143	150	157	165	172	179	186	193	200	208	215	222	229
6'0"	118	126	133	140	147	154	162	169	177	184	191	199	206	213	221	228	235
6'1"	122	129	137	144	151	159	166	174	182	189	197	204	212	219	227	235	242
6'2"	125	133	141	148	155	163	171	179	186	194	202	210	218	225	233	241	249
6'3"	129	137	145	152	160	168	176	184	192	200	208	216	224	232	240	248	256
6'4"	132	140	148	156	164	172	180	189	197	205	213	221	230	238	246	254	263

35	36	37	38	39	40	41	42	43	44	45	46	47	48	49	50	51	BMI
ounds)																	Height (feet/ inches)
ese						Extreme Obesity											
167	172	177	181	186	191	196	201	205	210	215	220	224	229	234	239	244	4'10"
173	178	183	188	193	198	203	208	212	217	222	227	232	237	242	247	252	4'11"
179	184	189	194	199	204	209	215	220	225	230	235	240	245	250	255	261	5'0"
185	190	195	201	206	211	217	222	227	232	238	243	248	254	259	264	269	5'1"
191	196	202	207	213	218	224	229	235	240	246	251	256	262	267	273	278	5'2"
197	203	208	214	220	225	231	237	242	248	254	259	265	270	278	282	287	5'3"
204	209	215	221	227	232	238	244	250	256	262	267	273	279	285	291	296	5'4"
210	216	222	228	234	240	246	252	258	264	270	276	282	288	294	300	306	5'5"
216	223	229	235	241	247	253	260	266	272	278	284	291	297	303	309	315	5'6"
223	230	236	242	249	255	261	268	274	280	287	293	299	306	312	319	325	5'7"
230	236	243	249	256	262	269	276	282	289	295	302	308	315	322	328	335	5'8"
236	243	250	257	263	270	277	284	291	297	304	311	318	324	331	338	345	5'9"
243	250	257	264	271	278	285	292	299	306	313	320	327	334	341	348	355	5'10"
250	257	265	272	279	286	293	301	308	315	322	329	338	343	351	358	365	5'11"
258	265	272	279	287	294	302	309	316	324	331	338	346	353	361	368	375	6'0"
265	272	280	288	295	302	310	318	325	333	340	348	355	363	371	378	386	6'1"
272	280	287	295	303	311	319	326	334	342	350	358	365	373	381	389	396	6'2"
279	287	295	303	311	319	327	335	343	351	359	367	375	383	391	399	407	6'3"
287	295	304	312	320	328	336	344	353	361	369	377	385	394	402	410	418	6'4"

* Adapted from National Institutes of Health, *Clinical Guidelines on the Identification, Evaluation, and Treatment of Overweight and Obesity in Adults: The Evidence Report*, NIH publication no. 98-4083, (September 1998), as cited on http://www.cdc.gov/healthy-weight/assessing/bmi/adult_bmi/index.html (accessed on August 23, 2012).

Now that you've calculated your "Right Weight," how do you get there? Before giving you the three-phase program for success, I am going to explain a few ground rules, just as I do at the beginning of every consultation with a new patient.

- First of all, remember that this diet is about you, that you are the one who will make it happen.

- Start the diet at your own pace, free of guilt and frustration. You have chosen to become slim and you should see that as something positive in your life.

- Accept the fact that any diet will require you to change your previous eating habits.

- Don't let yourself get discouraged. You have all the time you need. This isn't a race and it's the result that counts.

- Finally, don't focus on the stumbling blocks that can impede the success of a diet. You may be afraid that you'll be hungry, that you'll feel guilty if you snack or don't stick to the diet, that you'll cave in to temptation, or that it will take too long for the weight to come off. Learn to be patient with yourself and banish negative thoughts from your mind. You can do this.

CHAPTER 4

BEFORE YOU GET STARTED: DIET GUIDELINES

RULES FOR DIET SUCCESS

The following helpful tips are your keys to success with this diet plan.

1 Embrace your desire to lose weight

Write down what you wish to achieve and for whose sake you want to lose weight. This decision must be your own—you must be absolutely convinced that losing weight will be a tangible benefit to you. Tell your friends you're on a diet and ask for support by letting them know they will play a key role in your success. Reread your goals regularly, to help you get through the tough times and plateaus and stay motivated over time.

2 Define a realistic target weight

Don't try to lose too much, too quickly, by following a diet that is too restrictive for too long. And don't skimp. Eating a sufficient quantity of good food is the only way a diet is sustainable. The Right Weight formula (see page 56) will help you identify a reasonable and achievable goal.

3 Go at your own pace

The Parisian Diet is a three-phase solution, but not all of the phases are mandatory. The Café phase is intended as a brief jolt to stimulate the start of your weight-loss program, but you may find it too restrictive to maintain. In that case, you can start off with the Bistro phase. Adapt the diet according to your own desires. It might take a little longer for the weight to come off, but you need to be in control and you need to be able to stick with the diet. You can follow the Bistro phase for two to three weeks and the Gourmet phase for as long as you wish. In the end, it matters little whether it takes you two weeks or a month to lose your first ten pounds; what matters is getting there.

4 Allow yourself a treat

Frustration is the biggest challenge to successful dieting. Make a game out of your diet and plan your meals to give you something to look forward to. Nothing is strictly off limits. Allow yourself some "pleasure" foods that will serve as an occasional lifebuoy among the "obligatory" foods. We are omnivores, so you should eat a bit of everything and enjoy a varied diet. You will succeed in losing weight only if you respect your urges, cravings, and habits. Just remember that when you allow yourself to indulge such cravings, you will need to compensate beforehand and/or afterward. I'll explain how with the recovery plan (see page 268).

5 Redefine your habits

With this diet, you will rediscover the taste of food. Try different ways of preparing food rather than relying on what the food industry prepackages for you. Imagine, for example, chicken breast, cooked without fat but flavored with garlic or parsley. Instead of a simple tomato salad, treat yourself to gazpacho by blending the ingredients together. A diet should not be considered a brief hiatus in your life that is over once you reach your desired weight. Instead it should facilitate you to make significant changes to your daily routine, including your eating habits, to ensure that you will be able to maintain your new weight over the long term. Don't fool yourself into thinking that everything will be a breeze once you've finished dieting: in fact, it's after you've reached your weight-loss goal that everything starts. If you take advantage of this time to relearn the basics of food and nutrition—the taste of fruit and vegetables, how to cook without fat, how to select from the daunting variety of food choices available, and how to plan a meal so that you're not left feeling hungry—those skills will become second nature to you and you'll be able to incorporate them into your eating habits for life.

6 Find a balance and manage hunger

This diet is based on an increasing volume of food with a stable calorie intake, and on a balance of fiber, protein, and sugars. Protein is an essential component of our nutrition. You can't lose weight and improve your figure without it, because if you don't consume enough protein, the body will draw what it needs away from muscles and vital organs. Portioning your protein intake is essential, however, because when consumed in excess, proteins are converted into sugars and, eventually, into fat. Sugars are a source of glycogen, which stores energy in muscles, and this diet allows you to consume some sugars, primarily in the form of carbohydrates. The diet has been designed to feed your body the right balance of protein and sugar so each organ will get what it needs, leaving the body to draw energy from fat reserves, resulting in weight loss.

Unlimited rations of cooked and raw vegetables and fruits are intentionally introduced in the Bistro and Gourmet phases. This fills the stomach and intestine and provokes satiety—the feeling of being full— while at the same time increases the digestive process, which expends more energy and therefore enhances weight loss. Managing your hunger by eating a lot of fruit and vegetables will enable you to eat more and feel full without increasing your calorie intake.

7 Own your diet

To lose weight, you need to learn to manage food yourself. Standard diets where everything is imposed are never effective over the long term. That's why I give you a list of alternate sources of fiber, protein, and sugar, so you can make your own choices. For example, if a recipe calls for meat, but you're not in the mood for meat that day, you can replace it by choosing something from the list of equivalents (see pages 76–79). Similarly, you can swap one fruit or vegetable for another, based on what you want to eat that day.

8 Keep it simple

You can, of course, follow recipes, but you don't have to launch into elaborate cuisine using low-calorie ingredients. Leave that to those with plenty of time and to professional chefs. Instead use simple recipes like the ones in this book and experiment with different herbs, spices, and seasonings to delight your taste buds. Buy diet-friendly cooking equipment (nonstick pans, silicone molds, steamer, etc.).

9 Go easy on the eyes

The way you prepare food is of paramount importance. Many of us no longer eat much fruit. However, if you get creative with it—poach it, bake it, stew it, or whip up a fruit salad—it suddenly becomes more appealing. Don't neglect the presentation of food on your plate. The appearance of your meal can make eating all the more enjoyable.

10 Make healthy choices

When faced with multiple food options, it's important to make healthy choices. For example, two slices of toast with butter and jam contain 240 calories, but a slice of whole-wheat bread with a soft-boiled egg has only 180. A glass of diet soda has zero calories, whereas a non-diet version contains 70. Similarly, a portion of cheesecake contains 300 calories but a nonfat plain yogurt mixed with a fruit puree contains only about half that. And what a difference between a sausage hoagie (700 calories) and a ham and cheese club sandwich (300 calories)! Make sauces with less fat, use light cooking methods, and choose the most appropriate foods from the variety available.

11 Set your own schedule

We all have our preferred eating patterns. The French saying: "eat like a prince in the morning and a pauper in the evening," is not obligatory. While it is fundamental that you take an undistracted break of at least twenty to thirty minutes for each meal, you can time those meals according to your own rhythm. You can eat more at one meal and then less at another or you can swap something from one meal to another. For instance, if you don't like to eat first thing in the morning, have a mid-morning snack instead of breakfast. But if breakfast is an important meal for you, don't miss it. In this diet, you are not required to eat the menu items at a specific time of day. What is essential is that you stick to the items in the day's given menu over the course of the day. Your diet should suit your lifestyle and expectations. Always remember that it is important to be in control of your own life! You're in charge!

12 Don't change your lifestyle

Even if you are dieting, you should be able to participate in all of your usual activities. You just need solutions to help you cope with the desire to snack, or to know what foods to eat when you're faced with a business lunch or dinner with friends. See pages 261–264 for tips on how to stick to this diet in different situations when dining out.

13 Track your food intake

Post your weekly meal plans on your refrigerator so you don't leave any room for improvising. Keep a food journal of what you've eaten each day. You will notice that if your weight isn't going down, it's because what you've eaten has changed over the few days before weighing. A correctly followed diet will always produce results—not necessarily within two or three days, but certainly over the course of two weeks.

14 Weigh in and measure up

The bathroom scale is an important tool for monitoring a diet. Weigh yourself regularly, but don't make an obsession of doing so. You should weigh yourself once a week, first thing in the morning, before you've eaten but after urinating. Weight loss does not follow a consistent linear trajectory, so don't be discouraged if your weight hasn't varied. Also take four body measurements (thighs, hips, waist, and bust) often. They give you another way to evaluate the effectiveness of your diet, as it is possible to slim down without seeing a significant reduction in weight. Invest in a pedometer, to challenge yourself to increase your physical activity daily.

15 Reward yourself!

Give yourself a little treat, although not a food one, each time you make progress: a new pair of trousers, face cream, a massage … it's your choice! Believe in yourself!

Know Your Food Essentials

1 **Yogurt**

There is a slight difference in taste between whole yogurts and fat-free ones, but it's preferable to restrict yourself to the latter. Doing so will enable you to feel full without increasing your calorie intake. So-called fruit yogurts are simply fruit-flavored; while they rarely contain more than 12 percent fruit, there's no reason why you can't eat them as long as they don't contain sugar.

2 **Fresh or frozen vegetables**

You can use whatever vegetables are readily available. In terms of their nutritional value, fresh vegetables are no better for you than frozen or canned ones. It's a matter of choice and taste. It is much better to eat frozen vegetables than to go without them altogether. However, be wary of commercial preparations: check carefully that they don't contain added fats. Buying seasonal produce is always preferable.

3 **Vegetable soups**

Non-pureed soups, containing chunks of vegetables, are very satiating. Just avoid soups with added fats or carbohydrates. Instead, add extra flavor to soups by adding fennel or parsley. Zucchini is a good vegetable to add to thicken the soup.

4 **Fish and shellfish**

Tuna and salmon are higher in fat than other types of fish, but are fine if you keep serving sizes to the same portions as meat. Shellfish is a good seafood option that often gets overlooked. The allowance is four ounces, weighing edible parts, only, which represents approximately eight medium-sized shrimp.

5 Cheese

Restrict yourself to cheeses that contain less than 30 percent fat. This still leaves you with a wide selection. And you can certainly replace meat with cheese, which is a *très* French habit in the evening.

6 Eggs

Eggs should be eaten in moderation. The yolk is the most caloric part of the egg, and also the part that contains the most cholesterol. So it's preferable to eat only the whites, particularly if you are following a recovery plan after indulging (see page 268).

7 Drinks

Being adequately hydrated is vitally important, especially when dieting. Steer clear of drinks that contain sugar or alcohol. Instead, reach for mineral or tap water, tea, black coffee, and diet sodas. To make water more interesting, add a few drops of lemon, lime, or orange. Drinking the water you cook your vegetables in, if you like it, is an effective way to control your appetite.

Supermarket Survival Kit

Supermarket shopping is an essential part of our lives, but it is rife with traps for those who are trying to follow a healthy diet. So what can be done?

- Prepare a shopping list before you leave home and stick to it. Stock up on basic diet-friendly ingredients such as sweetener, herbs, spices, fat-free dairy products, eggs, fruit, vegetables.

- Go to the grocery store after you've eaten, so that you don't feel so tempted by the presence of food.

- Avoid going to the supermarket with your children, who will sometimes cause you to buy, whether from weakness on your part or pressure on theirs, more than you were planning to.

- Take the time to read the list of ingredients contained in your favorite products, to check that what you're buying matches the promises on the packaging. Don't forget that the first ingredient listed is the one that exists in the greatest quantity in the product. Be particularly vigilant regarding ready-made dishes to ensure that your "noodles with shrimp" does actually contain some shrimp along with the noodles.

- Look at the calorie content of the product, and always check whether the portion for which the nutrition facts are given corresponds to the quantity you plan to eat.

CHAPTER 5

KITCHEN ESSENTIALS

LIGHT COOKING METHODS

Diet prep starts in the kitchen. A monotonous diet will lead to frustration and loss of patience. In order to accustom your body to eating less, you need to vary the way you cook food. The following light cooking methods will add variety to mealtimes without extra fat and calories.

 Fruit and vegetables

- **Bake** in the oven wrapped in parchment paper or a sheet of aluminum foil
- **Boil** in a large amount of boiling water with salt
- **Broil** under the broiler
- **Dry-fry** in a very hot frying pan (with nonstick coating) or in a wok
- **Grill** on a flat-top grill or barbecue
- **Microwave** in a microwavable covered dish with a small amount of water added or wrapped in nonstick parchment paper
- **Steam** in a steamer or a pressure cooker
- **Stew** in a covered pan

Meat and fish

- **Bake** in the oven wrapped in parchment paper
  or a sheet of aluminum foil
- **Boil** in a large amount of boiling water with salt
  and a bouquet garni
- **Broil** under the broiler
- **Dry-fry** in a very hot frying pan (with nonstick coating)
  or in a wok
- **Grill** on a flat-top grill or barbecue
- **Microwave** wrapped in nonstick parchment paper
- **Steam** in a steamer or a pressure cooker

 Eggs

- **Bake** in the oven in a casserole or a ramekin
- **Boil** for 3 minutes for soft-boiled eggs, 5 minutes
  for medium-boiled, or 10 minutes for hard-boiled eggs
- **Microwave** in a microwavable ramekin or casserole
  for about 1 minute on average power
- **Poach** in boiling water with a few drops of vinegar
  for about 3 minutes
- **Scramble (or as an omelet)** in a hot frying pan (with nonstick
  coating) or with skim milk in a double-boiler

Carbohydrates/Starches

- **Boil** in a large amount of boiling water with salt
- **Simmer** rice with three times its volume of cold water in a hot pan (with nonstick coating) or a wok; cook until liquid is absorbed completely, stirring regularly
- **Soak** couscous in a salad bowl with one and a half times its volume of boiling water and a pinch of salt; cover and let rest until liquid is completely absorbed

Note: For potatoes, follow instructions for "Fruit and vegetables," page 69.

Spices and Herbs

Historically, people have depended on the aromatic properties of certain plants to enhance the flavor of their food. Spices and herbs are the key

Spices

Name	Form	Use with
Cinnamon	Ground Whole sticks	Fish (marinade) Fruit (salad, baked fruit dishes) Poultry (marinade) Rice Yogurt
Cloves	Ground Whole	Cabbage Meat (roast) Rice pilaf Soup, stock
Coriander	Ground Seeds	Baked dishes Stew
Cumin	Ground Seeds	Cabbage Fish fillet Lentils Potatoes Sauerkraut Vegetable soup
Curry	Ground Paste	Apples (oven-baked) Eggs Fish and Shellfish Lamb Pasta Rice Vegetables White meat

to avoiding monotony when dieting. They also stimulate healthy digestion. Here are some proven combinations to add pizzazz to your meals.

Name	Form	Use with
Nutmeg	Grated	Cabbage-based dishes Cheese-based dishes Fresh fruit: orange, pineapple, strawberry Lamb (ground meat) Potatoes Veal (ground meat) Vegetable gratin/puree
Paprika	Ground	Eggs Fish (marinade) Meat (marinade) Yogurt/cottage cheese for a spicy dip
Pepper	Whole peppercorns: Dried Ground	All dishes (freshly ground) Marinade
Saffron	Threads Powder	Fish Rice *Use with moderation in cooked dishes as it can make food taste bitter
Star Anise	Whole	Curry Soup
Vanilla	Extract Seeds Whole beans	Dairy products Fish (marinade) Fruit, dessert Poultry (marinade)

Herbs

Name	Form	Use with
Basil	Chopped Crushed	Eggs Pasta Poultry Soup Veal Vegetables (cooked), bell peppers, eggplant, salad greens, tomato (cooked or raw), zucchini *Loses its aroma when cooked
Bay Leaf	Dried Fresh	Soup Stew
Bouquet Garni (parsley, thyme, bay leaf)	Dried Fresh	Soup, stock Stew
Chervil	Dried Fresh	Eggs Fish Salad Sauces Soup
Chives	Fresh	Eggs Potatoes (steamed) Salad dressing Soup Yogurt
Cilantro	Fresh, chopped	Salad Soup (clear broth) Vegetables (cooked)
Dill	Fresh Ground Seeds	Cucumber and potato salad Fish (baked dishes) *Fresh: add to a cooked dish before serving *Ground/seeds: add when you start cooking

Name	Form	Use with
Mint	Fresh	Lamb
	Dried	Tea
Oregano	Dried	Meat (grilled/broiled)
		Tomato dishes (hot)
		Tomato sauce
		Vegetable gratin
Parsley	Fresh	Garnish
		Salad, salad dressing
		Sauces
		Soup
Rosemary	Fresh	Lamb (marinade, for grilling)
	Dried	Ratatouille
	Ground	White meat
Sage	Fresh	Fish
	Dried	Game
		Poultry
		Tea
Tarragon	Fresh	Eggs, omelet
	Dried	Salad dressing
	Ground	Tomato
		Vegetable soup (cream of)
		White meat
Thyme	Fresh	Meat (marinade)
	Dried	Soup
	Ground	Tomato/bell pepper dishes

Food Equivalents and Substitutes

I often mention "equivalent" foods that can be substituted for another ingredient in a recipe. The following list of food alternatives can be used to add variety to the recipes, or to replace a food you don't particularly enjoy or that is not readily available or in season.

 Protein (meat, fish, poultry, cheese)

4 oz. cooked chicken or turkey (white meat, no skin)

2 medium eggs

4 oz. cooked fish fillet (cod, flounder, haddock, halibut, salmon, trout, tuna—fresh, frozen, or canned in brine)

4 oz. shellfish, cleaned and shells removed (clams, crab, lobster, scallops, shrimp)

3 oz. lean ham, not marbled

4 oz. cooked lean meat: lean beef trimmed of fat (round, sirloin, flank steak); beef tenderloin; roast beef (chuck, rib); steak (T-bone, porterhouse, cubed); ground round; cooked lean pork; pork tenderloin; center pork loin chop; lean lamb chop; veal

4 oz. firm tofu

2 oz. hard cheese (cheddar, mozzarella, Swiss, Parmesan, American)

1 ½ cup (12 oz.) plain nonfat yogurt

1 cup (8 oz.) 2% milk fat cottage cheese

⅔ cup (6 oz.) 4% milk fat cottage cheese

Vegetables

2 cups (8 oz.) diced cucumber

2 cups (10 oz.) raw leafy greens (salad greens, sauerkraut, spinach)

1 cup (6 oz.) cooked leafy greens (Brussels sprouts, cabbage, celery, leeks, scallions)

1 cup (6 oz.) cooked vegetables (artichoke, asparagus, broccoli, cauliflower, eggplant, mushroom, pepper, pumpkin, radish, tomato)

½ cup (3 oz.) cooked diced starchy vegetables (yam, potato, sweet potato, green peas, plantain)

½ cup (3 oz.) cooked beans, lentils, peas (chickpeas, black-eyed peas, pinto beans, kidney beans)

Carbohydates/Starches

1 ½ tablespoons (¾ oz.) uncooked rice

⅓ cup (2 oz.) cooked rice

⅓ cup (1 ½ oz.) raw pasta

¾ cup (3 ½ oz.) cooked pasta

½ bagel

2 slices (2 oz.) bread

½ pita bread (6-inch diameter)

2 tablespoons (1 oz.) dry oats

½ cup (3 oz.) cooked whole oats

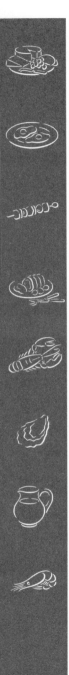

Milk and dairy products

½ cup (4 fl. oz.) 1% or 2% milk

1 cup (8 fl. oz.) skim milk

2 level tablespoons (½ oz.) powdered milk

¾ cup (6 oz.) plain low-fat yogurt

1 cup (8 oz.) plain nonfat yogurt

1 oz. hard cheese (American, cheddar, mozzarella, Parmesan, Swiss)

¼ cup (2 oz.) whole milk ricotta cheese

⅓ cup (3 oz.) part-skim ricotta cheese

⅓ cup (3 oz.) 4% milk fat cottage cheese

½ cup (4 oz.) 2% milk fat cottage cheese

⅔ cup (5 oz.) 1% milk fat cottage cheese

Fats

1 strip bacon

1 tablespoon (½ oz.) nonfat cream cheese, sandwich spread,
    or sour cream

1 teaspoon (¼ oz.) butter or margarine or vegetable oil

2 teaspoons (⅓ oz.) mayonnaise or peanut butter

6 nuts (almonds, cashews)

10 peanuts

10 olives

Fruit

1 small fruit / 1 slice / 1 cup (5 oz.) (chopped) of any fruit
1 ½ tablespoons (½ oz.) raisins
8 halves dried apricots
1 ½ dried figs
3 whole dates, pitted
3 prunes, dried, pitted
100% fruit juice:
  ½ cup (4 fl. oz.) apple juice
  ⅓ cup (2 ¾ fl. oz.) cranberry juice
  1 cup (8 fl. oz.) cranberry juice (lite or reduced calorie)
  ⅓ cup (2 ¾ fl. oz.) grape juice
  ½ cup (4 fl. oz.) grapefruit juice
  ½ cup (4 fl. oz.) orange juice
  ½ cup (4 fl. oz.) pineapple juice
  ⅓ cup (2 ¾ fl. oz.) prune juice

 Wine

Parisians enjoy wine—either as an aperitif before a meal or a glass with
a meal. A small 4 ¼ oz. (125 ml) glass can be substituted for a serving of fruit.

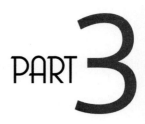

PART 3

THE THREE PHASES

GETTING STARTED

Diets that promise quick and easy solutions are alluring, but full of false promises that will keep you from achieving and sustaining your goal. Real success in weight loss can only be achieved by eating a well-balanced diet, based on medical expertise and adapted to modern life. And by doing so intelligently. This is really a simple method, you just need some determination to implement it.

And now it's time to get started. It's time for you to get going on a diet that you are going to enjoy. With the Parisian Diet, you are going to learn how to rebalance your eating habits. This diet ensures that you take in enough nutrients and that no food groups are off limits, so you won't get frustrated. It's not a revolutionary diet or a trendy one, but a simple process of learning—or relearning—how and what to eat that allows you to achieve a new healthy balance in your life. These practical, realistic guidelines also help you to stay healthy and maintain your new weight after dieting, which is a serious shortfall with other diets. At its core, this diet gives you all the tools you need to achieve a varied and healthy diet (for life!) and one in which pleasure is the key word!

The Parisian Diet diet offers, not imposes (the nuance is important), three phases:

- **Café phase** an optional and brief kick-start where you will lose up to one pound per day for up to a maximum of ten days,
- **Bistro phase** to follow for two to three weeks—you'll lose eight to eleven pounds,
- **Gourmet phase** where you will comfortably lose another eight to eleven pounds the first month, followed by an additional six to nine pounds every month thereafter for at least three months.

Each phase includes advice, recipes, and choices—*beaucoup*! But in order to understand them, you need to know the big picture. A diet is like a product label: it is important to start by reading the list of ingredients and the instructions carefully. You need to study, understand, and integrate them. Because, to be effective, a diet must not be swallowed in one gulp but rather assimilated and digested, like an exquisite (but not too large) glass of fine French wine.

CHAPTER 6

THE CAFÉ PHASE

In a Nutshell: How and When

T HE CAFÉ PHASE IS AN **optional** way to kick-start your weight loss.
It is designed for healthy adults who wish to lose the first few
pounds in a short time at the beginning of their diet, to give them the
incentive to continue. It is intentionally challenging and short term
because every pound you lose will give you the motivation to lose the
next and help you make the commitment to stick with the Parisian Diet
over time. However, this is a highly restrictive phase of the diet that
should only be undertaken by people in **good health** for a loss of up to
one pound per day over a **maximum of eight to ten days**. **Multivitamin
and magnesium supplements** are obligatory during the Café phase.

At any point during the Café phase, if you start to feel tired or that the
diet is too restrictive, you should move on to the Bistro phase.

The Café phase can also be used for a short period of **one to two
days** for a weight-loss boost of up to one pound per day if you hit
a plateau while following the Bistro (see pages 109–163) or Gourmet

(see pages 165–257) phases, or as part of the recovery plan (see page 268) to compensate for the occasional indulgence.

You should never go directly from the Café phase to normal eating without first following it up with the Bistro phase for a minimum of one week and then the Gourmet phase for a minimum of two weeks.

The French café is an unpretentious hub where locals start their day with the ritual of sipping an espresso while standing at the zinc bar. Gossip and small talk is exchanged, and then off they go to start their day. After lunch, it happens all over again. It's part of the fabric of life in France and is also an appropriate name for the first part of the diet. The Café phase is a quick start before moving on to the Bistro and Gourmet phases, and it includes a lot of liquids: smoothies, purees, soups, and beverages such as water, tea, and black coffee.

The nutritional principle is simple: consume a low-calorie diet that is extremely rich in minerals, vitamins, and trace elements. Because soups are very filling due to their high micronutrient content, they are effective at counteracting hunger pangs. Vegetable soups in particular are high in fiber and water and so low in calories. There is a famous French cabbage soup diet that made headlines; it was a hit: it went viral on the Internet, was photocopied and passed on all over the globe, and used by countless dieters as an effective way to lose weight quickly. What you may not know is that it originally came from a very rapid weight-loss diet that I developed for a French newspaper in the nineties and that originally consisted of many different varieties of soup.

The basis of that original diet, now combined into a range of carefully planned menus, is the optional Café phase of the Parisian Diet. Nevertheless, you must bear in mind that this is quite a restrictive phase, designed to be undertaken only by those in good health. You must take multivitamin and magnesium supplements and drink plenty of approved liquids (see page 111) throughout the day. These liquids should be sugar-free, but you may use sweeteners such as stevia or aspartame. If you are still hungry after a meal, you can add a plate of steamed vegetables, a green salad, endives, or other leafy greens seasoned with lemon juice.

Again, you should not go directly from this diet to normal eating without first following it up with the Bistro phase for one to two weeks and then the Gourmet phase for two to four weeks. I often have my patients follow this Café phase for one to two days if they are losing less than one pound per week. This helps them remain calm and stress-free during a plateau in their weight loss. And after a rather lax week, eating soup will rectify things.

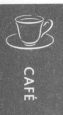

BREAKFAST

Banana and Pear Milk Shake

1 small pear (approximately 3 oz.), peeled, seeded, and diced

1 small banana (approximately 2 ¾ oz.), peeled

1 cup (8 fl. oz.) skim milk

1 teaspoon sweetener

Prep time: 3 min. / Ready in: 3 min.

Combine all the ingredients in a blender and blend until smooth and creamy. Serve chilled or with ice.

LUNCH

Zucchini and Cottage Cheese

1 medium zucchini (approximately 4 oz.), washed and diced

1 clove garlic, crushed

½ cup (5 oz.) 1% milk fat cottage cheese

Chives, chopped, to taste

Prep time: 2 min. / Cook time: 8 min. / Ready in: 10 min.

Heat zucchini and garlic in a dry nonstick frying pan over medium heat for about 8 minutes, stirring regularly until soft. Mix zucchini into cottage cheese and season with chives.

Nuts

6 walnut halves (approximately ½ oz.)

Cheese

1 oz. hard cheese (American, cheddar, Parmesan)

Leek Soup

3 large leeks (approximately 8 oz.), cleaned and thinly sliced

2 cups (16 fl. oz.) fat-free, reduced-sodium chicken broth

Black pepper

2 tablespoons fresh chives, minced

Prep time: 5 min. / Cook time: 35 min. / Ready in: 40 min. Serves 4

Put leeks and broth into a large soup pot. Cover and bring to a boil over high heat. Remove lid and reduce heat, simmer leeks until tender. Season with black pepper. Garnish with chives and serve.

Fruit

1 small apple (approximately 5 oz.), sliced

Cinnamon

Prep time: 2 min. / Ready in: 2 min.

Sprinkle cinnamon on apple slices, to taste. Serve.

CAFÉ

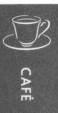
CLASSIC CAFÉ MENU 2

BREAKFAST

Apple–Yogurt Milk Shake

2 small apples (approximately 8 oz.), peeled, seeded, and diced

¾ cup (6 oz.) plain nonfat greek yogurt

1 teaspoon sweetener

¼ teaspoon vanilla extract

Prep time: 3 min. / Ready in: 3 min.

Combine all the ingredients in a blender and blend until smooth and creamy. Serve chilled or with ice.

LUNCH

Cod with Winter Squash

1 medium winter squash (approximately 2 cups/1 lb.), peeled and diced

1 medium onion, diced

3 oz. cod fillet

Salt and pepper

1 teaspoon finely chopped parsley

1 pinch curry powder

Nuts

6 almonds (approximately ½ oz.)

Prep time: 5 min. / Cook time: 30 min. / Ready in: 35 min.

Place winter squash and onion into a large soup pot, add water to cover top of squash. Cover and bring to a boil over high heat. Remove lid and reduce heat; simmer until squash is tender.

Steam the cod fillet for 10 minutes and season with salt, pepper, and parsley, to taste.

Drain excess water from squash, puree with blender, and season with curry powder, salt, and pepper, to taste.

Serve.

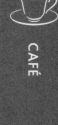

Seven Veggie Soup

1 cup (1 oz.) fresh spinach leaves, washed and trimmed

1 small zucchini (approximately 4 oz.), diced

2 small turnips (approximately 4 oz.), peeled and diced

2 large fresh tomatoes (approximately 4 oz.), seeded and diced

2 medium carrots (approximately ¼ lb.), peeled and sliced

1 small leek (approximately 3 ½ oz.), cleaned and thinly sliced

⅓ cup (3 ½ oz.) chopped green cabbage

2 cups (16 fl. oz.) fat-free vegetable broth

Salt and pepper

1 tablespoon finely chopped cilantro

Prep time: 10 min. / Cook time: 35 min. / Ready in: 45 min.

Serves 4

Put spinach, zucchini, turnip, tomatoes, carrots, leeks, cabbage, and vegetable broth into a large soup pot. Cover and bring to a boil over high heat. Remove lid and reduce heat; simmer until vegetables are tender. Season with salt and pepper, garnish with cilantro, and serve.

Fruit

1 orange (approximately 5 oz.)

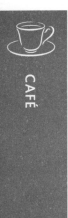

CLASSIC CAFÉ MENU 3

BREAKFAST

Kiwi Milk Shake

2 kiwis, peeled and halved
¾ cup (6 oz.) plain nonfat greek yogurt
1 teaspoon sweetener

Prep time: 3 min. / Ready in: 3 min.

Combine all the ingredients in a blender and blend until smooth and creamy. Serve chilled or with ice.

LUNCH

Curried Carrots and Yogurt

8 oz. baby carrots
½ teaspoon curry powder
½ teaspoon vanilla extract
1 ½ cups (12 oz.) plain nonfat yogurt
6 hazelnuts (approximately ¼ oz.), chopped

Prep time: 3 min. / Cook time: 10 min. / Ready in: 13 min.

Steam the carrots for 10 minutes. Mix curry powder and vanilla extract into yogurt. Mix carrots and yogurt together in a bowl. Garnish with the chopped hazelnuts and serve.

Cabbage Soup

3 cups (2 lb.) finely chopped green cabbage

2 large fresh tomatoes (approximately 12 oz.), seeded

Juice of ½ lemon

¾ cup (4 oz.) chopped onions

2 cups (16 fl. oz.) fat-free vegetable broth

2 small apples (approximately 10 oz.), peeled, seeded, and chopped

1 ½ tablespoons raisins

Salt and pepper

Prep time: 10 min. / Cook time: 25 min. / Ready in: 35 min.

Serves 4

Put green cabbage, tomatoes, lemon juice, onions, and vegetable broth into into a large soup pot. Cover and bring to a boil over high heat. Remove lid and reduce heat; let simmer until vegetables are tender. Toss in diced apples and raisins and simmer for 5 minutes. Season with salt and black pepper. Serve.

CAFÉ

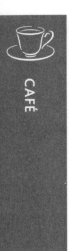
CLASSIC CAFÉ MENU 4

Breakfast

Berry Milk Shake

1 cup frozen mixed berries

¾ cup (6 oz.) plain nonfat
greek yogurt

1 teaspoon sweetener

Prep time: 3 min. / Ready in: 3 min.

Combine all the ingredients in a blender
and blend until smooth and creamy. Serve
chilled or with ice.

Lunch

Grilled Salmon with Sautéed Spinach

3 oz. salmon fillet

Dill, chopped, to taste

1 clove garlic, crushed

6 cups (6 oz.) spinach leaves,
washed and trimmed

1 tablespoon sliced almonds
(approximately ¼ oz.)

Parsley, chopped, for garnish

Prep time: 2 min. / Cook time: 15 min. / Ready in: 17 min.

Season the salmon fillet with dill, and bake,
broil, grill, or dry-fry for about 15 minutes,
until flaky. Dry-fry the garlic until soft; add
spinach with a little water and sauté for
about 5 minutes until wilted. Toast sliced
almonds until golden in a dry, nonstick
frying pan or toaster oven, then sprinkle
over cooked salmon. Garnish the meal with
chopped parsley. Serve.

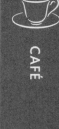

Butternut Soup

1 ½ cups (6 oz.) butternut squash, peeled and cut into cubes

2 cups (16 fl. oz.) fat-free vegetable broth

1 medium onion, peeled and chopped

Salt and black pepper

Ground nutmeg

Prep time: 10 min. / Cook time: 25 min. / Ready in: 35 min.

Serves 4

Put butternut squash, broth, and onion into a large soup pot. Cover and bring to a boil over high heat. Remove lid and reduce heat; simmer until squash is tender. Puree with a blender and season with salt, black pepper, and nutmeg to taste. Serve.

Fruit

1 cup canned fruit (8 ½ oz. packaged in light syrup), drained

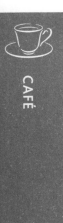
BREAKFAST

Tomato and Cucumber Smoothie

2 large fresh tomatoes (approximately 12 oz.), peeled and seeded

1 small cucumber (approximately 4 oz.), peeled and seeded

Juice of 1 lemon

½ grapefruit, peeled and sectioned

2 pinches celery salt

Prep time: 5 min. / Ready in: 5 min.

Combine all the ingredients in a blender and blend until smooth and creamy. Serve chilled or with ice.

LUNCH

Tilapia with Green Beans

3 oz. tilapia fillet

8 oz. green beans

2 shallots, chopped

Parsley, chopped

Juice of ½ lemon

Prep time: 5 min. / Cook time: 20 min. / Ready in: 25 min.

Broil, grill, or dry-fry the tilapia fillet for about 10 minutes until flaky. Sauté the green beans, chopped shallots, and parsley for 15 minutes in a dry, nonstick frying pan with ¼ cup water. Season the fillet with lemon juice and serve alongside the beans.

Tomato Soup

1 small onion, chopped

2 cloves garlic, crushed

¼ cup (2 oz.) canned tomato paste

2 cups (16 fl. oz.) fat-free vegetable broth

4 large fresh tomatoes (approximately 1 ½ lb.), coarsely chopped

2 teaspoons fresh thyme

Salt and pepper

Prep time: 5 min. / Cook time: 10 min. / Ready in: 15 min.

Serves 4

Add onion, garlic, tomato paste, and 1 tablespoon vegetable broth to a large saucepan; heat over medium heat, stirring until soft. Stir in the tomatoes with the rest of the broth, thyme, salt, and pepper. Cover and simmer until the vegetables are tender. Puree with a blender. Serve.

Fruit

1 small banana (approximately 2 ¾ oz.)

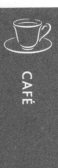

CLASSIC CAFÉ MENU 6

BREAKFAST

Mango and Banana Milk Shake

1 slice (5 oz.) mango, diced

1 small banana (approximately 2 ¾ oz.), peeled

1 cup (8 fl. oz.) skim milk

1 teaspoon sweetener

Prep time: 3 min. / Ready in: 3 min.

Combine all the ingredients in a blender and blend until smooth and creamy. Serve chilled or with ice.

LUNCH

Tomato and Sweet Red Pepper Provençal Flan with Cottage Cheese

1 small onion, chopped

1 clove garlic, crushed

3 medium fresh tomatoes (approximately 1 cup/10 oz.), peeled, seeded, and sliced

1 medium sweet red pepper (approximately ½ cup/4 oz.), seeded and chopped

Salt and black pepper

1 teaspoon fresh thyme

½ cup (4 oz.) 1% milk fat cottage cheese

Chives, chopped, to taste

1 tablespoon roasted pine nuts (approximately ¼ oz.)

Prep time: 5 min. / Cook time: 30 min. / Ready in: 35 min.

Preheat the oven to 375°F. Spread the onion and garlic on the bottom of the baking dish. Layer sliced tomatoes and red pepper alternately in the dish on top of the onion and garlic, fitting them in tightly. Season with salt, pepper, and thyme. Bake for 30 minutes, or until vegetables are tender. Serve with the cottage cheese, mixed with chopped chives and the pine nuts.

Cheese

1 oz. hard cheese (American, cheddar, Parmesan)

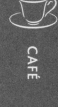

Carrot and Spinach Soup

1 cup (8 fl .oz.) fat-free vegetable broth

1 ½ cup (1 ½ oz.) spinach leaves, washed, trimmed, chopped

1 cup (8 oz.) chopped carrots

1 teaspoon ground cumin

Salt and pepper

Prep time: 5 min. / Cook time: 20 min. / Ready in: 25 min.

Serves 4

Put stock, spinach, carrots, and cumin into a large soup pot. Cover and bring to a boil over high heat. Remove lid and reduce heat; simmer until vegetables are tender. Season to taste with salt and pepper; serve.

Fruit

1 cup (7 oz.) fresh pineapple chunks (or 1 can [8 oz.] pineapple chunks packed in water, drained)

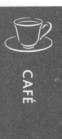
CLASSIC CAFÉ MENU 7

BREAKFAST

Fruit Yogurt

1 cup canned fruit (8 oz. packed
 in light syrup), drained
1 kiwi, peeled and diced
¾ cup (6 oz.) plain nonfat yogurt
1 teaspoon sweetener

Prep time: 3 min. / Ready in: 3 min.

In a bowl, add drained canned fruit, diced kiwi, yogurt, and sweetener. Mix and serve.

LUNCH

Grilled Scallops with Portobello Mushrooms

1 cup (3 oz.) portobello
 mushrooms, sliced
Salt and pepper
Parsley, chopped, to taste
3 oz. baby scallops
Paprika, to taste
1 tablespoon chopped walnuts
 (approximately ¼ oz.)

Prep time: 10 min. / Cook time: 15 min. / Ready in: 25 min.

Sauté the mushrooms in a dry, nonstick frying pan for 10 minutes. Season with salt, pepper, and parsley. Sauté the scallops seasoned with paprika for 5 minutes or until opaque in the center. Serve scallops, garnished with walnuts, alongside mushrooms.

Italian Vegetable Soup

1 cup fresh baby spinach leaves (approximately 1 oz.)

1 small zucchini (approximately 1 cup/4 oz.), cubed

1 small fennel bulb (approximately ½ cup/4 oz.), thinly sliced

1 cup (6 oz.) canned diced tomatoes

1 clove garlic, crushed

1 small sweet red pepper (approximately ½ cup/4 oz.), chopped

1 small onion, chopped

1 teaspoon fresh thyme

1 teaspoon oregano

2 cups (16 fl. oz.) fat-free vegetable broth

Salt and pepper

1 teaspoon chopped parsley

1 teaspoon chopped basil

Fruit

1 cup fresh watermelon (approximately 5 oz.), diced

Prep time: 10 min. / Cook time: 25 min. / Ready in: 35 min.

Serves 4

Put spinach, zucchini, fennel, diced tomatoes, garlic, red pepper, onion, thyme, oregano, and vegetable broth into a large soup pan. Cover and bring to a boil over high heat. Remove lid and reduce heat; simmer until vegetables are tender. Season with salt and pepper to taste. Garnish with parsley and basil, and serve.

CAFÉ

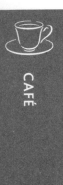
CLASSIC CAFÉ MENU 8

BREAKFAST

Citrus Fruit Salad

1 navel orange, peeled
  and sectioned
½ grapefruit, peeled
  and sectioned
½ lemon, peeled and sectioned
Juice of ½ lemon
½ teaspoon sweetener

Prep time: 10 min. / Ready in: 10 min.

Combine all ingredients and serve.

Yogurt

¾ cup (6 oz.) plain nonfat yogurt

LUNCH

Grilled Chicken and Broccoli

3 oz. chicken breast
Ground nutmeg
¾ cups (6 oz.) broccoli florets

Prep time: 5 min. / Cook time: 15 min. / Ready in: 20 min.

Grill, broil, or dry-fry the chicken until center is no longer pink, then season with nutmeg to taste. Steam the broccoli until tender. Serve.

Nuts

6 almonds (approximately ½ oz.)

Leek Soup

3 large leeks (approximately
  ½ lb.), cleaned and thinly sliced
2 cups (16 fl. oz.) fat-free,
  reduced-sodium chicken broth
Black pepper
2 tablespoons fresh chives,
  minced

*Prep time: 5 min. / Cook time: 35 min. / Ready in: 40 min.
Serves 4*

Put leeks and broth into a large soup pot.
Cover and bring to a boil over high heat.
Remove lid and reduce heat, simmer leeks
until tender. Season with black pepper.
Garnish with chives and serve.

or

Cabbage Soup
  (see page 93)

Fruit

1 cup (8 oz.) fresh berries

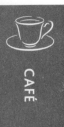
BREAKFAST

Kiwi–Mango Milk Shake

1 slice (5 oz.) mango, diced
1 kiwi, peeled and diced
¾ cup (6 oz.) plain nonfat yogurt
1 teaspoon sweetener
¼ teaspoon vanilla extract

Prep time: 3 min. / Ready in: 3 min.

Combine all the ingredients in a blender and blend until smooth and creamy. Serve chilled or with ice.

LUNCH

Vegetables with Cottage Cheese Dip

2 teaspoons chopped chives
2 shallots, chopped
1 cup (8 oz.) 1% milk fat cottage cheese
2 medium carrots
  (approximately 5 oz.)
¼ cucumber
  (approximately 5 oz.)
3 stalks celery

Prep time: 10 min. / Ready in: 10 min.

Mix the chives and shallots with the cottage cheese to make the dip. Chop the carrots, cucumber and celery into sticks for dipping. Serve.

Nuts

10 roasted unsalted peanuts
  (approximately 1 oz.)

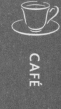

Asian Soup

1 cup (2 ½ oz.) chopped bok choy

1 cup (2 ½ oz.) chopped Chinese cabbage

1 clove garlic, crushed

¼ cup (2 oz.) thinly sliced sweet red pepper

4 shiitake mushrooms, chopped

1 teaspoon minced ginger root

2 cups (16 fl. oz.) fat-free vegetable broth

1 cup (2 ½ oz.) snow peas

1 tablespoon low-sodium soy sauce

1 tablespoon finely chopped cilantro

Prep time: 10 min. / Cook time: 20 min. / Ready in: 30 min.

Serves 4

Put bok choy, Chinese cabbage, garlic, red pepper, mushrooms, ginger, and broth into a large soup pan. Bring to a boil over high heat and then simmer until vegetables are tender. Toss in snow peas and simmer for 5 minutes. Stir in soy sauce and cilantro. Serve.

Fruit

1 small banana (approximately 2 ¾ oz.)

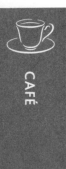

BREAKFAST

Apple and Pear Milk Shake

1 small pear (approximately
   5 oz.), peeled, seeded, and diced
1 small apple (approximately
   5 oz.), peeled, seeded, and diced
1 cup (8 fl. oz.) skim milk
1 teaspoon sweetener
1 pinch cinnamon

Prep time: 3 min. / Ready in: 3 min.

Combine all the ingredients in a blender and blend until smooth and creamy. Serve chilled or with ice.

LUNCH

Grilled Cod with Asparagus and Scallions

2 scallions, chopped
3 oz. cod fillet
Juice of ½ lemon
8–10 spears asparagus
2 tablespoons balsamic vinegar

Prep time: 10 min. / Cook time: 20 min. / Ready in: 30 min.

Dry-fry the scallions until transparent, add the cod, and cook until flaky, around 5 minutes. Season with lemon juice. Steam asparagus until tender. Dress the asparagus with balsamic vinegar and serve alongside the fish.

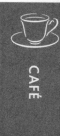

Leek Soup

3 large leeks (approximately
½ lb.), cleaned and thinly sliced

2 cups (16 fl. oz.) fat-free,
reduced-sodium chicken broth

Black pepper

2 tablespoons fresh minced
chives,

*Prep time: 5 min. / Cook time: 35 min. / Ready in: 40 min.
Serves 4*

Put leeks and broth into a large soup pot.
Cover and bring to a boil over high heat.
Remove lid and reduce heat, simmer leeks
until tender. Season with black pepper.
Garnish with chives and serve.

or

Cabbage Soup
(see page 93)

Fruit

1 peach (approximately 5 oz.)

CHAPTER 7

THE BISTRO PHASE

In a Nutshell: How and When

The Bistro phase allows for rapid weight loss of eight to eleven pounds in three weeks. It's fast because it's very restrictive. While it will decrease your appetite, it is difficult to uphold over time and is therefore designed for a maximum of three weeks before switching to the Gourmet phase for one month. After that period, if you have not yet reached your Right Weight, continue alternating weeks of the Bistro and Gourmet phases until you do.

Also use the Bistro phase:

- for seven days if you hit a weight loss plateau during the Gourmet phase,

- for two weeks if the Café phase is too difficult to maintain, or

- for a two to three day treatment if you gain a few pounds after reaching your Right Weight.

When following the Bistro phase, you should take multivitamin and magnesium supplements to avoid fatigue and cramps and drink plenty of liquids throughout the day.

Bistro Phase Ground Rules

Own It!

Feel free to customize recipes by swapping equivalent foods (see pages 76–79) according to your personal preferences.

At the beginning of a new phase in your diet, it's natural for you to want to lose weight fast: you're motivated to make the extra effort to get quick results. The Bistro phase will help you to slim down quickly while still consuming a sufficient amount of food to prevent you from feeling overly tired. Nevertheless, this phase is not designed to be followed for a long period of time; after two to three weeks you need to

---

Sample Daily Allowance

Breakfast

- Black coffee, tea, or herbal tea in unlimited quantities, with sweetener and 2 tablespoons (1 fl. oz.) of skim milk, if desired.

- ¾ cup (6 oz.) nonfat plain yogurt with sweetener if desired, or 1 cup (8 fl. oz.) skim milk, or equivalent protein.

Mid-morning

- Black coffee, tea, or herbal tea in unlimited quantities, with sweetener and 2 tablespoons (1 fl. oz.) of skim milk, if desired.

Lunch

- Raw vegetables or salad in unlimited quantities, seasoned with unsweetened lemon juice, vinegar, mustard, shallots, onions, garlic, herbs, and spices, if desired.

- 3 oz. lean meat, fish, or 2 medium eggs, or equivalent protein (see page 76), cooked without fat.

- 1 cup (6 oz.) non-starchy vegetables, boiled or steamed without fat.

---

alternate it with menus from the Gourmet phase so you retain your initial enthusiasm and don't give up on the diet.

For breakfast, you can have a nonfat plain yogurt without sugar, but you can add sweetener if you wish, or instead of yogurt select an equivalent food from the list provided (see pages 76–79). For example, you could have a glass of milk instead or another nonfat dairy product.

In addition, I recommend that you drink unlimited quantities, at any time, of water, as well as black coffee, tea, or herbal tea—with sweetener instead of sugar, as desired—or, drink nonfat vegetable broth, which is rich in minerals and vitamins and suppresses the appetite.

- ¾ cup (6 oz.) nonfat plain yogurt with sweetener, or 1 cup (8 fl. oz.) skim milk, or equivalent protein.

- 1 piece (5 oz.) of fruit.

Afternoon
- Black coffee, tea, or herbal tea in unlimited quantities, with sweetener and 2 tablespoons (1 fl. oz.) of skim milk, if desired.

Dinner
- Raw vegetables or salad in unlimited quantities, seasoned with unsweetened lemon juice, vinegar, mustard, shallots, onions, garlic, herbs, and spices, if desired.

- 3 oz. lean meat, fish, or 2 medium eggs, or equivalent protein (see page 76), cooked without fat.

- Non-starchy vegetables, boiled or steamed without fat, in unlimited quantities.

- ¾ cup (6 oz.) nonfat plain yogurt with sweetener if desired or 1 cup (8 fl. oz.) skim milk, or equivalent protein.

- 1 piece (5 oz.) of fruit.

In the following menus, the dressings and dips for raw vegetables do not contain any fat, but you may replace the ones on pages 170–173 with a maximum of two tablespoons (1 fl. oz.) low-calorie salad dressing (choose one that contains less than 300 calories per 3 ½ fl. oz.). Feel free to use seasonings, herbs, lemon juice, and nonfat bouillon cubes to flavor vegetables and other nonfat foods. Finally, enjoy the pleasure of losing weight. This will keep you motivated during the brief period you are on this phase of the diet. Do not add fat or oil when cooking vegetables, fish, or meat.

Throughout the Bistro phase, lunch and dinner recipes can be transposed or you can split to allow you more, but smaller, meals throughout the day, such as a mid-morning or afternoon snack.

The results obtained by following a strict diet over a long period of time are no better than those obtained by alternating the same strict diet with another, easier, one. You can therefore alternate menus from the Bistro phase with the menus from the Gourmet phase.

I've also varied the types of cheese and vegetables to highlight the importance of a range of choice for certain food groups. They provide the freshness and variety that prevent the diet from becoming too bland, and help to adapt your taste buds. For cheese, keep in mind that it will be more economical to consume the same cheese for several days until you have finished the package, so choose one that you like!

The Bistro phase consists of three styles of menu options that can all be alternated throughout the week:

- **Classic Bistro Menu Options** (see pages 114–133) provide a good variety of recipes to keep your motivated.

- **Quick Bistro Menu Options** (see pages 134–143) prevent boredom by offering recipes with a quick and easy twist. As with jogging, it helps to vary the pace! The first menus offer sweeter recipes, with more carbs in the form of fruit. They also feature more substantial breakfasts, while the evening meal is more frugal. These recipes are aimed to please those sweet-toothed dieters who struggle with the lack of sugar in other diets. And it's especially geared to people who have little time to spare, as the meals are very quick to prepare.

- **Carb-Lover Bistro Menu Options** (see pages 144–163) allow you to eat carbohydrates and starches as part of your evening meal, which can ease hunger pangs in the night and help you sleep. Be aware, however, that these menus should be mixed with regular menus from throughout this Bistro phase, and the carb menu options should not be followed for more than ten days straight.

BREAKFAST

Yogurt

¾ cup (6 oz.) plain nonfat yogurt
  (with sweetener as desired)

LUNCH

Cod Fillet with Julienned Vegetables

1 medium carrot, peeled and cut into very thin sticks

1 medium zucchini, cut into very thin sticks

1 stalk celery, cut into very thin sticks

½ onion, finely sliced

3 oz. cod fillet (fresh or frozen)

Salt and pepper

Few leaves parsley, chopped

Juice of ½ lemon

¼ cup (2 oz.) 1% milk fat cottage cheese

Prep time: 5 min. / Cook time: 30 min. / Ready in: 35 min.

Preheat oven to 375°F. Place half of the carrot, zucchini, celery, and onion onto a square of parchment paper, top with the cod fillet, then cover with the remaining vegetables. Season with salt and pepper, parsley, and a drizzle of lemon juice. Close tightly and bake for about 30 minutes. Remove from parchment paper and serve with cottage cheese.

Asparagus with Yogurt Dressing

6 spears asparagus

1 teaspoon balsamic vinegar

⅓ cup (3 oz.) plain nonfat yogurt

Prep time: 5 min. / Cook time: 10 min. / Ready in: 15 min.

Boil or steam the asparagus until tender. Mix balsamic vinegar with yogurt, drizzle over asparagus. Serve.

Fruit

½ grapefruit

BISTRO: CLASSIC

Heart of Palm Salad

1 cup hearts of palm (10 oz., drained)

2 tablespoons Herb Vinaigrette (see below)

Prep time: 2 min. / Ready in: 2 min.

Dress hearts of palm with herb vinaigrette and serve.

Herb Vinaigrette

1 bunch fresh herbs of your choice (parsley, dill, chervil, chives, basil, tarragon...), chopped

¾ cup (6 oz.) plain nonfat yogurt

Dash of lemon juice or vinegar

1 shallot, chopped

Salt and pepper, to taste

Prep time: 5 min. / Ready in: 5 min.

Serves 4

Mix ingredients together. Keep unused dressing refrigerated.

Turkey with Collard Greens

1 clove garlic, crushed

3 oz. turkey breast

1 small bunch collard greens

Prep time: 5 min. / Cook time: 15 min. / Ready in: 20 min.

Broil, grill, or dry-fry the garlic with the turkey breast until the center of the meat is opaque. Steam the collard greens for 10 minutes. Serve.

Cheese

1 slice (1 oz.) Swiss cheese

Fruit

1 cup stewed fruit (sugar-free)

BISTRO: CLASSIC

BREAKFAST

Yogurt

¾ cup (6 oz.) plain nonfat yogurt
(with sweetener as desired)

LUNCH

Aida Salad

¼ cup green peas
1 medium tomato, diced
¼ cup (3 oz.) diced bell pepper
¼ cup chopped artichoke hearts
1 teaspoon water
1 teaspoon vinegar
Juice of 1 lemon
1 teaspoon Dijon mustard
Salt and pepper

Prep time: 10 min. / Ready in: 10 min.

Mix the vegetables together. Make the dressing by mixing water, vinegar, lemon juice, mustard, and salt and pepper. Pour dressing over vegetables and serve.

Roast Beef and Parsnips with Cottage Cheese

3 oz. lean roast beef
1 teaspoon Dijon mustard
1 cup (6 oz.) chopped parsnips
Few sprigs parsley, chopped
½ cup (4 oz.) 1% milk fat cottage
cheese

Prep time: 5 min. / Cook time: 20 min. / Ready in: 25 min.

Preheat the oven to 375°F. Roast the beef for around 10 minutes or as desired and garnish with mustard. Steam the parsnips until tender and sprinkle with parsley. Serve with cottage cheese.

Fruit

1 apple

Radish Salad with Ham and Broccoli

¾ cup (6 oz.) broccoli florets, steamed

1 small bunch (approximately 13) radishes

2 tablespoons Herb Vinaigrette (see page 115)

2 slices (2 oz.) lean ham

Prep time: 10 min. / Cook time: 10 min. / Ready in: 20 min.

Steam the broccoli until tender. Slice the radishes and dress with herb vinagrette; serve with the ham and broccoli.

Cheese

1 oz. hard cheese (American, cheddar, Parmesan)

Fruit

1 orange

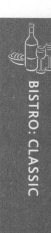

BISTRO: CLASSIC

BREAKFAST

Yogurt

¾ cup (6 oz.) plain nonfat yogurt
(with sweetener as desired)

LUNCH

Carrot and Celery Salad

2 medium carrots

1 stalk celery

2 tablespoons Herb Vinaigrette
(see page 115)

Prep time: 10 min. / Ready in: 10 min.

Grate the carrots and celery and dress with the herb vinagrette. Serve.

Veal and Mozzarella Melt

3 oz. veal cutlet

¼ cup (1 oz.) grated mozzarella cheese

1 cup (3 oz.) green beans

1 clove garlic, crushed

½ cup pureed tomatoes

Prep time: 10 min. / Cook time: 15 min. / Ready in: 25 min.

Grill, broil, or dry-fry the veal for about 5 minutes or until opaque in center. Cover with mozzarella and heat until the cheese melts. In a saucepan, heat the green beans with the garlic in the pureed tomatoes for 10 minutes. Serve.

Fruit

1 cup canned fruit (8 oz. packed in light syrup), drained

Beet and Apple Slaw

Prep time: 5 min. / Ready in: 5 min.

1 tablespoon lemon juice

1 tablespoon cider vinegar

Salt and pepper

1 cup (8 oz.) grated raw beet

1 apple, grated

1 tablespoon chopped parsley

In a bowl, mix together the lemon juice, cider vinegar, and salt and pepper. Add grated beets and apple. Toss well. Sprinkle with chopped parsley and serve.

Arugula Omelet

Prep time: 2 min. / Cook time: 8 min. / Ready in: 10 min.

2 medium eggs

½ cup (¾ oz.) arugula

¼ cup (2 oz.) part-skim ricotta cheese

Whisk the eggs, mix in the arugula and ricotta cheese, and cook in a nonstick frying pan for 8 minutes. Serve.

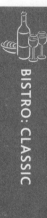

BISTRO: CLASSIC

BREAKFAST

Yogurt

¾ cup (6 oz.) plain nonfat yogurt
   (with sweetener as desired)

LUNCH

Cucumber Slices with Chives and Lemon Juice

½ cucumber, peeled
1 tablespoon chopped chives
½ tablespoon lemon juice

Prep time: 5 min. / Ready in: 5 min.

Slice the cucumber and season with chives and lemon juice. Serve.

Scallops with Capers

2 cups (16 fl. oz.) water
1 carrot, peeled and sliced
1 onion, chopped
1 bouquet garni
Salt and pepper
3 oz. scallops
2 cloves garlic
4 shallots, chopped
Small bunch parsley, chopped
3 tablespoons apple cider vinegar
2 tablespoons capers

Prep time: 5 min. / Cook time: 12 min. / Ready in: 17 min.

Put the water, carrot, onion, bouquet garni, and salt and pepper into a large saucepan; bring to a boil over high heat. Wash the scallops and poach for 5 minutes in the broth. Remove scallops with a slotted spoon, drain, and keep warm. In a non-stick frying pan, dry-fry the garlic, shallots, and parsley. together with the carrots and onion from the broth, for 5 minutes. Add the broth with the vinegar and capers, and simmer for 2 minutes. Drizzle the sauce over the scallops and serve.

Roasted Zucchini with Basil

2 small zucchini, sliced into rounds

1 handful basil, chopped

Salt and pepper

Prep time: 5 min. / Cook time: 20 min. / Ready in: 25 min.

Preheat oven to 400°F. Layer a nonstick baking dish with zucchini and bake for 20 minutes. Season with fresh basil and salt and pepper. Serve.

Yogurt

¾ cup (6 oz.) plain nonfat yogurt (with sweetener as desired)

Fruit

1 cup (7 oz.) fresh pineapple chunks

DINNER

Beef with Cauliflower Salad

3 oz. beef steak

1 teaspoon ketchup

1 cup (8 oz.) cauliflower florets

1 stalk celery, chopped

2 tablespoons Herb Vinaigrette (see page 115)

Prep time: 10 min. / Cook time: 15 min. / Ready in: 25 min.

Coat beef with ketchup and grill, broil, or dry-fry for about 5 minutes, or as desired. Steam the cauliflower and celery for 10 minutes until tender; dress with the herb vinaigrette. Serve.

Cheese

1 slice (1 oz.) Emmental or Swiss cheese

Baked Apple

1 apple, cored

Prep time: 3 min. / Cook time: 30 min. / Ready in: 33 min.

Preheat oven to 350°F. Add a tablespoon of water to a baking dish and bake the apple for about 30 minutes or until tender. Serve.

BREAKFAST

Yogurt

¾ cup (6 oz.) plain nonfat yogurt
(with sweetener as desired)

LUNCH

Cabbage Salad

1 cup (2 oz.) shredded red
cabbage
2 tablespoons Herb Vinaigrette
(see page 115)

Prep time: 2 min. / Ready in: 2 min.

Dress cabbage with herb vinagrette, serve.

Apple Pork and Carrots

3 oz. lean pork
5 baby carrots
Pinch ground cumin
¼ cup (2 oz.) applesauce
with no added sugar

Prep time: 5 min. / Cook time: 15 min. / Ready in: 20 min.

Grill, broil, or dry-fry the pork for 8 minutes
or until opaque in center. Add applesauce
and heat through. Meanwhile, steam carrots
for about 10 minutes until slightly tender
and season with ground cumin. Serve.

Frosted Orange

1 orange
⅓ cup (3 oz.) plain nonfat yogurt
¼ cup (2 oz.) 1% milk fat cottage
cheese
2 teaspoons powdered sweetener

Prep time: 10 min. / Cook time: 1 hour 30 min. / Ready in: 1 hour 40 min.

Cut off the top ¾ inch of the orange like a
hat. Carefully scoop out the flesh with a
knife and a spoon. Place the peel "bowl"
and "hat" in the freezer.
Remove and discard the seeds and pith
from the pulp. Mix the pulp with the
yogurt, cottage cheese, and sweetener.
Freeze for 30 minutes; then pour into the
frosted peel "bowl." Return to the freezer
for an hour. Put the hat on the frosted
orange, and serve immediately.

BISTRO: CLASSIC

Artichoke Salad

1 cup artichoke hearts

1 tablespoon balsamic
vinegar

Prep time: 2 min. / Ready in: 2 min.

Dress the artichoke with the balsamic
vinegar, serve.

Roast Beef and Provençal Tomatoes

3 oz. beef

2 medium tomatoes

1 tablespoon herbes de Provence

Prep time: 10 min. / Cook time: 40 min. / Ready in: 50 min.

Preheat oven to 400°F. Grill, broil, or roast
the beef for 10 minutes. Cut the tomatoes
in half and place, cut side up, on a baking
sheet. Sprinkle with herbes de Provence
and season. Cook in the oven for about
30 minutes until tender. Serve with
the beef.

Cheese

¼ cup (2 oz.) part-skim ricotta
cheese

Fruit

1 cup canned fruit (8 oz. packed
in light syrup), drained

BISTRO: CLASSIC

BREAKFAST

Yogurt

¾ cup (6 oz.) plain nonfat yogurt
(with sweetener as desired)

LUNCH

Asparagus with Lemon Juice

6 spears asparagus
Lemon juice, to taste

Prep time: 5 min. / Cook time: 10 min. / Ready in: 15 min.

Boil or steam the asparagus for 10 minutes or until tender. Serve with a drizzle of lemon juice.

Portuguese-style Baked Fish Fillet and Green Beans

2 onions, chopped
½ cup (1 ½ oz.) sliced
  mushrooms
2 large tomatoes, sliced
3 oz. cod fillet
Salt and pepper
2 tablespoons (1 oz.) fat-free
  vegetable broth
1 cup (3 oz.) green beans

Prep time: 10 min. / Cook time: 30 min. / Ready in: 40 min.

Preheat oven to 350°F. Place the chopped onion, mushrooms, and half of the tomatoes in a nonstick ovenproof dish. Lay the cod fillets on top. Add salt and pepper, and then cover with the remaining tomatoes. Drizzle with vegetable broth. Bake for 30 minutes.
Meanwhile, steam the green beans for 10 minutes. Serve.

Yogurt

¾ cup (6 oz.) plain nonfat yogurt
(with sweetener as desired)

Fruit

1 apple

BISTRO: CLASSIC

Carrot and Celery Sticks with Herb Vinaigrette

1 medium carrot

1 stalk celery

2 tablespoons Herb Vinaigrette (see page 115)

Prep time: 5 min. / Ready in: 5 min.

Chop the carrot and celery into sticks, dress with herb vinaigrette, and serve.

Lamb Skewers with Cauliflower and Feta

3 oz. lamb

½ teaspoon dried oregano

1 cup (8 oz.) cauliflower florets

1 teaspoon Dijon mustard

¼ cup (2 oz.) reduced-fat feta cheese, cut into cubes

Prep time: 10 min. / Cook time: 20 min. / Ready in: 30 min.

Chop the lamb into chunks and thread onto skewers. Season with oregano, and grill or broil for 10 minutes. Steam the cauliflower for 10 minutes. Serve together, with mustard garnish and feta.

Fruit

1 cup (7 oz.) fresh pineapple chunks

BISTRO: CLASSIC

BREAKFAST

Yogurt

¾ cup (6 oz.) plain nonfat yogurt
(with sweetener as desired)

LUNCH

Artichoke Salad

1 cup artichoke hearts

2 tablespoons Herb Vinagrette
(see page 115)

Prep time: 2 min. / Ready in: 2 min.

Dress artichoke hearts with herb vinaigrette and serve.

Grilled Flank and Vegetables

3 oz. lean beef flank steak

1 cup (8 oz.) eggplant

2 medium tomatoes

Few leaves basil

Prep time: 5 min. / Cook time: 25 min. / Ready in: 30 min.

Grill, broil, or dry-fry the beef for 5 minutes. Chop the eggplant and tomatoes and simmer them together for about 20 minutes with the basil. Serve.

Yogurt

¾ cup (6 oz.) plain nonfat yogurt
(with sweetener as desired)

Apple Meringue

1 apple, peeled and chopped

Vanilla extract, ground cinnamon, or lemon juice, to taste

½ egg white

½ teaspoon powdered sweetener

Prep time: 5 min. / Cook time: 25 min. / Ready in: 30 min.

Preheat oven to 400°F. Heat apples and chosen flavoring with ¼ cup (2 fl. oz.) water in a saucepan on high heat for 10 minutes. Meanwhile, beat egg white until stiff then add the sweetener gradually, folding in gently so the white doesn't collapse. Place the applesauce in a ramekin, top with the egg white, and heat in the oven for about 15 minutes until browned.

Sliced Cucumber

½ cup (3 ¾ oz./1 small)
cucumber, sliced

2 tablespoons Herb Vinagrette
(see page 115)

Prep time: 2 min. / Ready in: 2 min.

Dress cucumber slices with vinaigrette;
serve.

Grilled Pork
and Spinach

3 oz. pork chop

2 large handfuls spinach

½ sweet onion, sliced

Prep time: 5 min. / Cook time: 10 min. / Ready in: 15 min.

Grill, broil, or dry-fry the pork chop for
5 minutes or until center is opaque. Wash
the spinach and shake to remove most of
the water. Cook, covered, with the sweet
onion for 5 minutes until wilted. Serve.

Cheese

½ cup (4 oz.) 1% milk fat cottage
cheese

Fruit

Small bunch of grapes
(approximately 17 grapes)

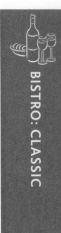

BISTRO: CLASSIC

BREAKFAST

Yogurt

¾ cup (6 oz.) plain nonfat yogurt
(with sweetener as desired)

LUNCH

Green Salad

1 large handful (½ oz.) Romaine
lettuce
2 tablespoons Herb Vinaigrette
(see page 115)

Prep time: 2 min. / Ready in: 2 min.

Dress lettuce with herb vinaigrette and
serve.

Chicken Breast and Leek Parcel

3 leeks, washed and chopped
Salt and pepper
3 oz. chicken breast
1 slice tomato
Juice and zest of 1 lemon
Few leaves tarragon, chopped
1 teaspoon fat-free chicken stock
diluted in ½ cup (4 fl. oz.) of
water

Prep time: 5 min. / Cook time: 30 min. / Ready in: 35 min.

Preheat oven to 400°F. Steam the leeks for
10 minutes until softened, and season.
Dry-fry the chicken breast in a hot nonstick skillet for about 2 minutes each
side to brown. Place a bed of leeks onto a
parchment paper square. Place the chicken
breast on the leeks, add the tomato, and
sprinkle with lemon juice. Season. Add the
tarragon and lemon zest to the chicken
stock and pour over the chicken. Seal
the parchment parcel and bake for about
15 minutes or until the chicken is cooked
through. Serve.

Yogurt

¾ cup (6 oz.) plain nonfat yogurt
(with sweetener as desired)

Fruit

1 kiwi

Dinner

Tomato–Cucumber Salad

¼ cup (3 oz.) chopped tomatoes
⅓ cup (2 oz.) cucumber, chopped
2 tablespoons lemon juice
Pepper, to taste

Prep time: 2 min. / Ready in: 2 min.

Mix together and serve.

Roast Beef Steak and Zucchini

3 oz. lean beef steak
1 cup (1 small) sliced zucchini
1 teaspoon dried oregano
Salt and pepper

Prep time: 5 min. / Cook time: 10 min. / Ready in: 15 min.

Season the beef steak with salt, pepper, and oregano; grill, broil, or dry-fry for 10 minutes. At the same time, steam the zucchini. Serve.

Cheese

½ cup (4 oz.) 1% milk fat
  cottage cheese

Fruit

1 orange

BREAKFAST

Yogurt

¾ cup (6 oz.) plain nonfat yogurt
(with sweetener as desired)

LUNCH

Green Salad

3 handfuls (3 oz.) lettuce
2 tablespoons Herb Vinaigrette
(see page 115)

Prep time: 2 min. / Ready in: 2 min.

Dress lettuce with herb vinagrette and serve.

Grilled Chicken with Pumpkin Puree

3 oz. chicken thigh
1 clove garlic, sliced
Few sprigs rosemary
1 cup (4 oz.) cubed pumpkin
Salt and pepper

Prep time: 10 min. / Cook time: 20 min. / Ready in: 30 min.

Season the chicken thigh with garlic and rosemary and grill, broil, or dry-fry for 10 minutes. Meanwhile, steam the pumpkin for 20 minutes, season with salt and pepper, and mash into a puree. Serve.

Yogurt

¾ cup (6 oz.) plain nonfat yogurt
(with sweetener as desired)

Fruit

1 orange

Green Beans

1 cup (3 oz.) green beans, trimmed
1 tablespoon balsamic vinegar
1 teaspoon Dijon mustard

Prep time: 2 min. / Cook time: 10 min. / Ready in: 12 min.

Steam green beans for 10 minutes until tender. Mix vinegar and mustard together into a dressing and toss with the beans. Serve

Grilled Tuna and Eggplant

1 medium eggplant
3 oz. fresh tuna steak
1 teaspoon mixed herbs
2 teaspoons lemon juice

Prep time: 5 min. / Cook time: 30 min. / Ready in: 35 min.

Preheat the oven to 400°F. Prick the eggplant and bake it for 30 minutes until tender. Meanwhile, season the tuna with herbs and lemon juice and grill, broil, or dry-fry for 5 minutes. Serve with green beans from previous recipe.

Cheese

½ cup (4 oz.) 1% milk fat cottage cheese

Fruit

1 pear

BISTRO: CLASSIC

BISTRO: CLASSIC

BREAKFAST

Yogurt

¾ cup (6 oz.) plain nonfat yogurt
  (with sweetener as desired)

LUNCH

Veal with Zucchini in Tomato Sauce

3 oz. veal cutlet

For the tomato sauce:

1 onion, finely chopped

1 clove garlic, crushed

1 tablespoon olive oil

4 large tomatoes (approximately
  1 ½ lb.), peeled and seeded

Salt and pepper

1 small zucchini, sliced

1 cup (2 oz.) baby corn

1 teaspoon chopped basil

Prep time: 10 min. / Cook time: 30 min. / Ready in: 40 min.

Preheat the oven broiler to 375°F. Broil the veal for 30 minutes or until tender. Meanwhile, make the tomato sauce: Sauté the onion and garlic in the olive oil until transparent. Add the tomatoes, salt, and pepper. Simmer for 15 minutes then blend with a blender. Add the zucchini and baby corn to the tomato sauce; cook for 10 minutes. Serve veal with the tomato–zucchini mixture, garnish with basil.

Cheese

½ cup (4 oz.) 1% milk fat
  cottage cheese

Fruit

3 clementines

Grated Zucchini Salad

1 cup (4 oz.) grated zucchini
2 tablespoons Herb Vinaigrette
(see page 115)

Prep time: 2 min. / Ready in: 2 min.

Mix together and serve.

Sirloin Steak with Beet and Chives

3 oz. sirloin steak
½ cup (4 oz.) cubed raw beet
1 tablespoon chopped chives
1 teaspoon ketchup

Prep time: 5 min. / Cook time: 20 min. / Ready in: 25 min.

Grill, broil, or dry-fry the steak for 5 minutes, or as desired. Steam the beet for 15 minutes. Garnish beets with chives and serve with steak and ketchup, if desired.

Cheese

1 slice (1 oz.) American cheese

Fruit

1 slice (5 oz.) mango

BISTRO: CLASSIC

BREAKFAST

Soft-boiled Egg and Cottage Cheese

1 medium egg
Drop of vinegar
2 slices (2 oz.) whole grain bread
½ cup (4 oz.) 1% milk fat cottage cheese

Prep time: 5 min. / Cook time: 3 min. / Ready in: 8 min.

Bring water to a boil in a saucepan. Add a drop of vinegar and 1 egg. Toast bread. Once water begins to boil again, cook egg for 3 minutes, then rinse with cold water. Serve egg and toast alongside cottage cheese.

LUNCH

Oven-baked Cod with Broccoli Puree

3 oz. cod fillet
2 teaspoons lemon juice
½ cup (4 oz.) broccoli florets

Prep time: 5 min. / Cook time: 15 min. / Ready in: 20 min.

Preheat oven to 400°F. Season the cod with lemon juice and bake for about 10 minutes until just cooked through. Meanwhile, boil or steam the broccoli for 5 minutes or until very tender; mash. Serve.

Fruit

1 cup (4 oz.) grapes

DINNER

Mango Yogurt

1 ½ cups (12 oz.) plain nonfat yogurt
1 slice (5 oz.) mango, diced

Prep time: 3 min. / Ready in: 3 min.

Mix together in a bowl and serve.

BISTRO: QUICK

BREAKFAST

Ricotta Crispbreads

2 reduced-fat crispbread crackers
(about 1 oz.)

¼ cup (2 oz.) part-skim ricotta
cheese

Prep time: 3 min. / Ready in: 3 min.

Top crackers with ricotta and serve.

Yogurt

¾ cup (6 oz.) plain nonfat yogurt
(with sweetener as desired)

LUNCH

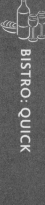

Beef Patty with Corn

3 oz. lean ground beef patty

½ cup corn kernels

1 tablespoon chopped parsley

Prep time: 5 min. / Cook time: 10 min. / Ready in: 15 min.

Grill, broil, or dry-fry the beef patty for
10 minutes. Meanwhile, heat the corn and
garnish with parsley. Serve.

Fruit

1 apple

DINNER

Vanilla–Pear Yogurt

¾ cup (6 oz.) plain nonfat yogurt

1 pear, diced

2 drops vanilla extract

Prep time: 3 min. / Ready in: 3 min.

Mix together in a bowl and serve.

Cheese

1 oz. hard cheese (American,
cheddar, Parmesan)

BREAKFAST

Cheddar Toast

2 slices (2 oz.) whole grain bread, toasted

1 slice (1 oz.) cheddar cheese

Prep time: 3 min. / Ready in: 3 min.

Top toast with cheddar, and serve.

Yogurt

¾ cup (6 oz.) plain nonfat yogurt (with sweetener as desired)

LUNCH

Ham and Grilled Eggplant on Toast

1 medium eggplant, sliced

2 slices (2 oz.) lean ham

2 slices (2 oz.) whole grain bread, toasted

Prep time: 5 min. / Cook time: 10 min. / Ready in: 15 min.

Grill, broil, or dry-fry the eggplant for 10 minutes or until tender. Serve with slices of ham on the toasted bread.

Fruit

3 clementines

DINNER

Apple Yogurt

1 ½ cups (12 oz.) plain nonfat yogurt

½ cup (4 oz.) cinnamon applesauce with no added sugar

Prep time: 3 min. / Ready in: 3 min.

Mix together in a bowl and serve.

BREAKFAST

Salmon Bagel with Cottage Cheese

1 whole grain bagel

2 oz. smoked salmon

½ cup (4 oz.) 1% milk fat cottage cheese

Prep time: 3 min. / Ready in: 3 min.

Toast bagel, top with salmon, and serve alongside cottage cheese.

LUNCH

Steamed Garlic–Cilantro Carrots with Soft-boiled Eggs

2 medium carrots

1 clove garlic, crushed

Few sprigs cilantro

2 medium eggs

Prep time: 10 min. / Cook time: 15 min. / Ready in: 25 min.

Steam the carrots for 15 minutes and season with crushed garlic and cilantro. Soft-boil the eggs and serve together.

Fruit

½ grapefruit

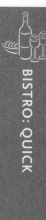

BISTRO: QUICK

DINNER

Lychee Yogurt

¾ cup (6 oz.) plain nonfat yogurt

⅓ cup (2 ½ oz.) lychees in light syrup, drained

Prep time: 3 min. / Ready in: 3 min.

Mix together in a bowl and serve.

Cheese

1 oz. hard cheese (American, cheddar, Parmesan)

BREAKFAST

Toasted Peanut Butter

2 teaspoons peanut butter
2 slices (2 oz.) whole grain bread, toasted

Prep time: 3 min. / Ready in: 3 min.

Spread peanut butter on toasted bread. Serve.

Milk

1 cup (8 fl. oz.) skim milk

LUNCH

Cucumber, Crab, and Tomato Salad

½ medium cucumber, diced
3 oz. crab meat
2 medium tomatoes, diced
1 tablespoon balsamic vinegar

Prep time: 10 min. / Ready in: 10 min.

Mix the cucumber, crab meat, and tomatoes and season with balsamic vinegar. Serve.

Fruit

1 kiwi

DINNER

Fruity Cottage Cheese

1 cup (8 fl. oz.) 1% milk fat cottage cheese
1 cup canned fruit (8 oz. packed in light syrup), drained

Prep time: 3 min. / Ready in: 3 min.

Mix together in a bowl and serve.

BREAKFAST

Cheddar Crispbreads

2 reduced-fat crispbread crackers (about 1 oz.)

1 slice (1 oz.) Swiss cheese

Prep time: 3 min. / Ready in: 3 min.

Top crackers with Swiss cheese and serve.

Milk

1 cup (8 fl. oz.) skim milk

LUNCH

Sautéed Shrimp with Zucchini

2 medium zucchini

3 oz. shrimp

1 clove garlic, crushed

Small handful parsley, chopped

Prep time: 10 min. / Cook time: 15 min. / Ready in: 25 min.

Dice the zucchini and steam for 10 minutes. Sauté the shrimp with the garlic and parsley for 5 minutes. Serve.

Fruit

½ grapefruit

DINNER

Pineapple Yogurt

1 ½ cups (12 oz.) plain nonfat yogurt

1 cup (7 oz.) fresh pineapple chunks

Prep time: 3 min. / Ready in: 3 min.

Mix in bowl and serve.

BISTRO: QUICK

Breakfast

Ricotta Omelet

1 medium egg

¼ cup (2 oz.) part-skim ricotta cheese

Prep time: 2 min. / Cook time: 5 min. / Ready in: 7 min.

Beat egg with ricotta; heat in nonstick frying pan for 5 minutes, and serve.

Yogurt

¾ cup (6 oz.) plain nonfat yogurt (with sweetener as desired)

Lunch

Curried Haddock with Vegetables

½ cup (3 ½ oz.) potatoes, diced

½ cup (4 oz.) chopped leeks

3 oz. fresh haddock fillet

½ teaspoon curry powder

Prep time: 10 min. / Cook time: 20 min. / Ready in: 30 min.

Preheat oven to 400°F. Boil the potatoes for 15 minutes. Steam the leeks for 10 minutes. Meanwhile, season the haddock with curry powder and bake in a parchment paper parcel for about 10 minutes until just cooked through. Serve.

Fruit

1 small banana

Dinner

Cinnamon Milk

2 cups (16 fl. oz.) skim milk

2 teaspoons ground cinnamon, or to taste

2 drops vanilla extract

1 teaspoon powdered sweetener, optional

Prep time: 3 min. / Cook time: 2 min. / Ready in: 5 min.

Warm the milk in a saucepan over medium heat for 2 minutes and add cinnamon, vanilla extract, and sweetener if desired.

Fruit

1 diced apple

BREAKFAST

Cottage Cheese and Toast

2 slices (2 oz.) whole grain bread, toasted

½ cup (4 oz.) 1% milk fat cottage cheese

Prep time: 3 min. / Ready in: 3 min.

Serve together.

Yogurt

¾ cup (6 oz.) plain nonfat yogurt (with sweetener as desired)

LUNCH

Roast Beef and Vegetables

3 oz. beef roast

1 cup (3 ¼ oz.) sliced mushrooms

1 clove garlic, crushed

Small handful parsley, chopped

½ cup canned kidney beans, drained

Prep time: 10 min. / Cook time: 15 min. / Ready in: 25 min.

Preheat oven to 400°F. Roast the beef for about 15 minutes, according to taste. Meanwhile, heat the mushrooms in a little water in a nonstick frying pan with garlic and parsley. Serve with kidney beans.

Fruit

1 orange

DINNER

Honey Yogurt

¾ cup (6 oz.) plain nonfat yogurt

2 teaspoons honey

Prep time: 2 min. / Ready in: 2 min.

Mix together and serve.

Cheese

1 oz. hard cheese (American, cheddar, Parmesan)

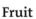

BISTRO: QUICK

BREAKFAST

Crispbreads with Ham and Cheddar

2 reduced-fat crispbread crackers (about 1 oz.)
2 thin slices (1 ½ oz.) lean ham
1 slice (1 oz.) cheddar cheese

Prep time: 3 min. / Ready in: 3 min.

Top crispbreads with ham and cheddar; serve.

LUNCH

Tuna Salad

3 oz. canned tuna in water
1 cup shredded lettuce
2 medium tomatoes, sliced
½ cup baby artichoke hearts
1 tablespoon balsamic vinegar

Prep time: 10 min. / Ready in: 10 min.

Mix ingredients together and season with balsamic vinegar.

Fruit

1 cup (7 oz.) fresh pineapple chunks

DINNER

Fruity Yogurt

1 ½ cups (12 oz.) plain nonfat yogurt
1 cup canned fruit (8 oz. packed in light syrup), drained

Prep time: 3 min. / Ready in: 3 min.

Mix together and serve.

BISTRO: QUICK

BREAKFAST

Turkey Bagel with Cottage Cheese

1 whole grain bagel, toasted

2 slices (2 oz.) turkey ham

½ cup (4 oz.) 1% milk fat cottage cheese

Prep time: 3 min. / Ready in: 3 min.

Top bagel with turkey ham. Serve with cottage cheese.

LUNCH

Grilled Chicken and Vegetables

3 oz. chicken breast

1 tablespoon soy sauce

1 cup (4 oz.) bean sprouts

½ cup (1 oz.) baby corn

Few sprigs cilantro, chopped

Prep time: 10 min. / Cook time: 10 min. / Ready in: 20 min.

Season the chicken breast with soy sauce and grill, broil, or dry-fry for 10 minutes. Meanwhile, steam the bean sprouts and baby corn for 10 minutes; garnish with cilantro. Serve.

DINNER

Banana Yogurt

1 small banana

½ teaspoon ground cinnamon, or less to taste

¾ cup (6 oz.) plain nonfat yogurt

Prep time: 3 min. / Ready in: 3 min.

Mash the banana and mix with cinnamon and yogurt.

Cheese

1 oz. hard cheese (American, cheddar, Parmesan)

BISTRO: QUICK

BREAKFAST

Toasted Peanut Butter

2 teaspoons peanut butter

2 slices (2 oz.) whole grain bread, toasted

Prep time: 3 min. / Ready in: 3 min.

Spread peanut butter on toasted bread. Serve.

Milk

1 cup (8 fl. oz.) skim milk

LUNCH

Roast Beef and Squash

3 oz. sliced lean roast beef

1 cup (4 oz.) squash, cubed

Fruit

1 apple

Prep time: 5 min. / Cook time: 15 min. / Ready in: 20 min.

Preheat oven to 400°F. Roast beef for 10 minutes or as desired. Meanwhile, steam or boil the squash for 15 minutes and mash. Serve.

Raisin Couscous

¼ cup dry couscous
(approximately 1 cup cooked)

⅓ cup (2 ¾ fl. oz.) fat-free
vegetable broth

1 tablespoon raisins

Prep time: 5 min. / Cook time: 5 min. / Ready in: 10 min.

Cook the couscous in the vegetable broth
for 5 minutes and add raisins. Serve.

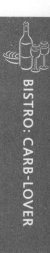

BISTRO: CARB-LOVER

BREAKFAST

Cottage Cheese and Toast

2 slices (2 oz.) whole grain bread, toasted

½ cup (4 oz.) 1% milk fat cottage cheese

Prep time: 3 min. / Ready in: 3 min.

Serve toast with cottage cheese.

Yogurt

¾ cup (6 oz.) plain nonfat yogurt (with sweetener as desired)

Fruit

1 small banana

LUNCH

Egg Salad

2 medium eggs

2 medium tomatoes

½ medium cucumber

Large handful shredded lettuce

1 tablespoon balsamic vinegar

Prep time: 5 min. / Cook time: 5 min. / Ready in: 10 min.

Boil the eggs for 5 minutes. Dice the tomatoes and cucumber, mix with the lettuce, and season with balsamic vinegar. Rinse hard-boiled egg under cold water, remove shell, and dice. Mix ingredients together and serve.

Fruit

1 orange

Spaghetti in Tomato Sauce

2 ounces dry or 1 ½ cups (7 oz.)
    cooked spaghetti

⅓ cup Tomato Sauce
    (see page 173)

Fruit

1 kiwi

Prep time: 5 min. / Cook time: 10 min. / Ready in: 15 min.

Boil spaghetti for about 5 minutes or according to package instructions, meanwhile heat tomato sauce. Top spaghetti with sauce and serve.

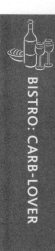

BISTRO: CARB-LOVER

BREAKFAST

Crispbreads

2 reduced-fat crispbread crackers
(about 1 oz.)

2 teaspoons jam

1 slice (1 oz.) American cheese

Prep time: 3 min. / Ready in: 3 min.

Spread crackers with jam and top with cheese. Serve.

Yogurt

¾ cup (6 oz.) plain nonfat yogurt
(with sweetener as desired)

LUNCH

Tilapia with Scallions and Oyster Sauce

2 tablespoons oyster sauce

1 teaspoon soy sauce

1 teaspoon sesame oil

½ teaspoon rice vinegar

3 oz. tilapia (or other fish) fillets,
cut into 2-inch pieces

1 stalk scallion, cut into 1-inch
lengths

Fruit

1 small banana

Prep time: 24 min. / Cook time: 6 min. / Ready in: 30 min.

In a large bowl, mix together the oyster sauce, soy sauce, ½ teaspoon sesame oil, and rice vinegar. Add the fish, cover, and let sit for 20 minutes.

Heat another ½ teaspoon sesame oil in a nonstick frying pan over medium-high heat until a piece of scallion dropped in the pan sizzles. Add the fish, distributing it evenly around the pan. Cook without stirring for 3 minutes. Add the scallion and stir gently. Continue to heat, stirring occasionally and gently, until the thickest part of a piece of fish is opaque throughout, 2–3 minutes more. Serve.

Soy Rice

Scant ½ cup (2 ½ oz.) brown rice

1 tablespoon soy sauce, to taste

1 tablespoon chopped cilantro

Prep time: 3 min. / Cook time: 20 min. / Ready in: 23 min.

Boil the brown rice in 1 cup (8 fl. oz.) water for 20 minutes, drain well. Season with soy sauce and cilantro. Serve.

Fruit

1 cup canned fruit (8 oz. packed in light syrup), drained

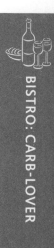

BISTRO: CARB-LOVER

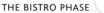

BREAKFAST

Turkey–Ricotta Toast

2 slices (2 oz.) whole grain bread, toasted

¼ cup (2 oz.) part-skim ricotta cheese

2 slices (2 oz.) sliced turkey

Prep time: 3 min. / Ready in: 3 min.

Top the toast with ricotta cheese and turkey. Serve.

Fruit

1 pear

LUNCH

Grilled Chicken with Green Beans

3 oz. chicken breast

1 cup (3 oz.) green beans

1 tablespoon chopped parsley

½ cup (4 oz.) applesauce with no added sugar

Prep time: 10 min. / Cook time: 15 min. / Ready in: 25 min.

Grill, broil, or dry-fry the chicken breast for 5 minutes. Steam the green beans for 10 minutes and garnish with parsley. Serve with applesauce.

Paprika Cornmeal

Prep time: 2 min. / Cook time: 10 min. / Ready in: 12 min.

¼ cup dry cornmeal

1 teaspoon paprika

Cook the cornmeal according to package instructions, but without fat, and season with paprika. Serve.

Fruit

1 cup (5 oz.) fresh watermelon chunks

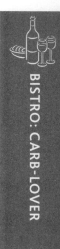

BISTRO: CARB-LOVER

BREAKFAST

Bagel with Eggs

1 medium egg

½ whole grain bagel, toasted

½ cup (4 oz.) 1% milk fat cottage cheese

Prep time: 3 min. / Cook time: 5 min. / Ready in: 8 min.

Boil egg as desired. Serve with bagel and cottage cheese.

Fruit

½ grapefruit

LUNCH

Grilled Shrimp with Zucchini

3 oz. shrimp

1 teaspoon fresh grated ginger

Few sprigs basil

1 medium zucchini

Prep time: 10 min. / Cook time: 15 min. / Ready in: 25 min.

Grill or dry-fry the shrimp with ginger and basil for 5 minutes. Grill or dry-fry the zucchini for 10 minutes. Serve.

Fruit

1 cup (4 oz.) grapes

Spicy Kidney Bean and Corn Salad

1 cup canned kidney beans, drained

½ cup cooked corn

1 tablespoon hot chili sauce, or to taste

Fruit

1 slice (5 oz.) mango

Prep time: 5 min. / Cook time: 10 min. / Ready in: 15 min.

In a saucepan, heat the kidney beans, corn, and chili sauce for 10 minutes over medium heat. Serve.

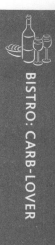

BISTRO: CARB-LOVER

BREAKFAST

Cereal

½ cup unfrosted whole grain cereal

1 cup (8 fl. oz.) skim milk

2 teaspoons honey

Prep time: 2 min. / Ready in: 2 min.

Mix ingredients together in a bowl and serve.

Nuts

6 almonds (approximately ½ oz.)

LUNCH

Turkey Patty with Mixed Greens

½ cup (1 ½ oz.) green beans

½ cup (2 oz.) baby sugar snap peas

3 oz. lean ground turkey patty

1 clove garlic, crushed

Prep time: 10 min. / Cook time: 15 min. / Ready in: 25 min.

Steam the vegetables for 10 minutes. Grill, broil, or dry-fry the turkey patty and garlic for 5 minutes. Serve.

Fruit

1 cup (4 oz.) blueberries

Quinoa

¼ cup dry quinoa

Fruit

1 cup canned fruit (8 oz. packed
in light syrup), drained

Prep time: 5 min. / Cook time: 20 min. / Ready in: 25 min.

Rinse and soak quinoa in water for
5 minutes. Drain and cook according
to package instructions. Serve.

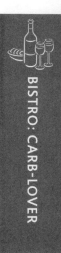

BISTRO: CARB-LOVER

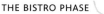

BREAKFAST

Pancake

1 frozen pancake

2 teaspoons maple syrup

½ cup (4 oz.) 1% milk fat cottage cheese

Prep time: 3 min. / Ready in: 3 min.

Heat pancake, top with maple syrup, and serve with cottage cheese.

Milk

1 cup (8 fl. oz.) skim milk

LUNCH

Sardines

3 oz. sardines, drained

Vegetable Soup

1 cup (8 fl. oz.) fat-free vegetable soup (less than 100 calories per serving)

Cook time: 5 min. / Ready in: 5 min.

Heat soup in microwave or saucepan. Serve.

Fruit

3 clementines

Pasta

¼ cup uncooked pasta spirals

1 tablespoon Tomato Sauce
  (see page 173)

Prep time: 1 min. / Cook time: 8 min. / Ready in: 9 min.

Boil pasta for about 8 minutes until cooked. Heat tomato sauce. Top pasta with sauce and serve.

Baked Apple

1 apple, cored

Cinnamon

Prep time: 3 min. / Cook time: 30 min. / Ready in: 33 min.

Preheat oven to 350°F. Add a tablespoon of water to a baking dish and bake the apple for about 30 minutes or until tender. Season with cinnamon and serve.

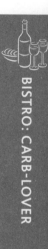

BISTRO: CARB-LOVER

BREAKFAST

Bacon and Eggs

2 slices Canadian bacon

1 medium egg

2 slices (2 oz.) whole grain bread, toasted

Prep time; 3 min. / Cook time: 12 min. / Ready in: 15 min.

Dry-fry bacon, set aside on papertowels to drain excess fat. Beat egg, pour into dry nonstick pan, and scramble. Serve.

Juice

1 cup (8 fl. oz.) orange juice

LUNCH

Ham Salad

2 slices (2 ½ oz.) lean ham, diced

¼ cup pickles, diced

1 stalk celery, chopped

½ cup (4 oz.) carrots, diced

½ cup (1 oz.) baby corn, diced

Prep time: 10 min. / Ready in: 10 min.

Combine all the ingredients and serve.

Fruit

1 cup (4 oz.) grapes

Curried Lentils

¾ cup dry red lentils (for
  1 ½ cups cooked lentils)

1 teaspoon curry powder

Prep time: 5 min. / Cook time: 20 min. / Ready in: 25 min.

Rinse lentils and soak in water for
5 minutes. Cook over high heat for
20 minutes, or until soft. Season with curry
powder, and serve.

Fruit

1 cup canned fruit (8 oz. packed,
  in light syrup), drained

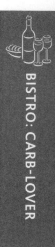

BISTRO: CARB-LOVER

BREAKFAST

Cereal

½ cup (4 oz.) unfrosted whole
grain cereal

1 cup (8 fl. oz.) skim milk

Prep time: 2 min. / Ready in: 2 min.

Mix together in a bowl and serve.

Cheese

½ cup (4 oz.) 1% milk fat cottage
cheese

Fruit

1 diced apple

LUNCH

Sirloin Steak with Bamboo Shoots and Broccoli

3 oz. sirloin steak

2 teaspoons soy sauce

1 cup sliced bamboo shoots

1 cup (8 oz.) broccoli florets

Prep time: 10 min. / Cook time: 15 min. / Ready in: 25 min.

Season the steak with soy sauce and grill,
broil, or dry-fry for 5 minutes; slice finely.
Steam bamboo shoots and broccoli for
10 minutes. Serve.

Fruit

1 cup (4 oz.) raspberries

Corn Salad

1 cup cooked chickpeas
½ cup cooked corn kernels
Few sprigs basil, chopped
Few sprigs cilantro, chopped
1 tablespoon lemon juice

Fruit

1 kiwi

Prep time: 5 min. / Ready in: 5 min.

Combine all the ingredients and serve.

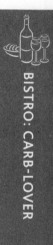

BISTRO: CARB-LOVER

BREAKFAST

Waffle

1 frozen waffle
2 teaspoons honey
½ cup (4 oz.) 1% milk fat
  cottage cheese

Prep time: 3 min. / Ready in: 3 min.

Heat waffle, top with honey, and
serve alongside cottage cheese.

Milk

1 cup (8 fl. oz.) skim milk

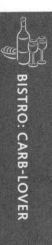

LUNCH

Sautéed Scallops
and Mushrooms

3 oz. baby scallops
1 clove garlic, crushed
Few springs parsley,
  chopped
1 cup (3 ¼ oz.) sliced
  mushrooms

Prep time: 10 min. / Cook time: 10 min. / Ready in: 20 min.

Sauté the scallops in a nonstick skillet with
the garlic, parsley, and mushrooms
for 10 minutes. Serve.

Fruit

1 orange

Japanese Noodles

4 oz. Japanese noodles (such as Ramen), (to yield ½ cup, cooked)

2 teaspoons soy sauce

2 teaspoons hot chili sauce

Fruit

1 slice (5 oz.) mango

Prep time: 1 min. / Cook time: 10 min. / Ready in: 11 min.

Boil Chinese noodles for 5 minutes or as desired. Garnish with soy sauce and hot chili. Serve.

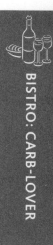

BISTRO: CARB-LOVER

Chapter 8

THE GOURMET PHASE

In a Nutshell: How and When

The Gourmet phase is designed for pure enjoyment and consists of delicious menus that make it easy to stay on course long term. On average, you can expect to lose eight to eleven pounds the first month, and, depending on the individual, six to nine pounds for each subsequent month.

During the Gourmet phase, if your weight loss stagnates, follow the Café or Bistro phases for a few days to lose a couple of pounds.

Gourmet Phase Ground Rules

Gourmet Menu Options

In addition to the overall guidelines for the Gourmet phase, I have included four special styles of menu options to help those of you who need inspiration or who are struggling to restore the necessary dimension of pleasure into the diet—the menus will help you make it through until you reach your goal weight and actually let you enjoy foods, such as potatoes, pasta, and bread, that many other diets eschew as taboo.

- **Classic Gourmet Menus** (see pages 174–201) provide a good variety of recipes—they can be followed consecutively or interspersed with the following menu options.

- **Gourmet Potato Menus** (see pages 202–215): Most diets eliminate certain foods that are vilified as the source of fat and weight gain. At the top of the list of these banished foods—enemy number one, according to some—is the potato. However, potatoes have a lot going for them, nutritionally: a 3 ½ oz. serving of potatoes contains 90 calories, 19 g complex carbohydrates, 30 mg magnesium, 380 mg potassium, and 1 mg iron. Low in cellulose, the potato is an easily digestible food that is also very filling. Because it is easy to digest, it prevents increased body temperature, which aids sleep and thus makes it an ideal food to eat as part of an evening meal. So how has the potato gotten itself such a bad name? From the fact that we've become accustomed to eating it with fat in the form of butter, cream, and deep-fried oil. If you incorporate potatoes without these harmful additions, there's no problem. The gourmet potato menus include delicious and nutritious potato-based recipes that you can either enjoy for a full week straight or mix up with daily menus from elsewhere in this Gourmet phase.

- **Gourmet Pasta Menus** (see pages 216–229): Pasta is another typically "forbidden" food in many diets, again, with no good reason. Energy-wise, regular pasta contains 355 calories per 3 ½ oz., 12.5% protein, 1.2% fat, 73.5% carbohydrate, and 4% fiber. It's easy to create a pasta-based diet, provided you balance all meals. The gourmet pasta menus can be used for a week-long pasta fiesta, or you can intersperse them with menu options from throughout this Gourmet phase.

- **Gourmet Sandwich Menus** (see pages 230–243): A common misconception is that dieting and bread are incompatible. On average, bread contains 250 calories per 3 ½ oz., 8% protein, and 50% complex carbohydrates. An important source of vitamin B, it is also rich in magnesium—0.3% in white bread and 0.9% in whole-wheat bread—as well as in copper. It contains no fat—except in the case of some commercially manufactured bread—and is very filling. The gourmet sandwich menus celebrate the humble sandwich. For added pleasure, nothing tastes better than fresh bread bought warm from a local bakery or the bakery section of your supermarket.

- **Gourmet Vegetarian Menus** (see pages 244–257): Throughout all three phases of the Parisian Diet, you can easily replace meat ingredients to create a vegetarian option using the protein food equivalents (see page 76). Vegetarian diets are rich in fiber and are therefore excellent for digestion. On a vegerarian diet, women run the risk of iron deficiency, but this can be avoided by eating plenty of lentils and fortified multigrain bread and/or breakfast cereal, or even by taking iron supplements.

French cuisine is famous for its sauces and dressings, but many traditional sauces are too rich in cream and butter. Instead, I have included a number of healthy sauces and marinades that will offer flavorful bases for your recipes.

- **Vinaigrette, Dressing, and Sauce Recipes** (see pages 170–173) make several servings and all will keep for several days in the refrigerator. The dressings may be used instead of one teaspoon of oil from a menu recipe, as desired.

Own It!

You can tailor your own personal diet plan: the daily menus can be used in any order you desire. Different days can be swapped around and mixed with those from the special Gourmet menu options that appear later in the chapter. And for further customization, you can follow the recipe suggested in the menu for each meal, or choose an option from the sample daily allowance (see pages 168–169). As long as you consume all of the items (or their equivalents) in one full menu each day, you can even feel free to invert mealtimes, having dinner for breakfast and vice versa if you so desire.

The most important thing to keep in mind when customizing the following menus is to stay faithful to the given quantities, because it's the balance between the portions and food groups that makes the difference between a healthy diet and one that is too rich. Unless otherwise specified in the list of food equivalents and substitutions (see pages 76–79), you should always stick to the following portion sizes:

4 oz. lean meat or fish

¾ cup (6 oz.) plain nonfat yogurt

⅔ cup (5 oz.) 1% milk fat cottage cheese

1 oz. hard cheese

1 piece (5 oz.) of fruit

It's important to stay hydrated while dieting, so drink unlimited quantities of water, as well as sugar-free drinks such as black coffee, tea, herbal teas, diet sodas, and even vegetable stock, which is an excellent appetite suppressant. To make vegetable stock, simply simmer vegetables in water for a long time to allow their minerals and vitamins

SAMPLE DAILY ALLOWANCE

Breakfast

- Black coffee, tea, or herbal tea in unlimited quantities, with sweetener and 2 tablespoons (1 fl. oz.) of skim milk, if desired.

- 1 slice (1 oz.) bread with 2 level teaspoons (⅓ oz.) butter or margarine *or* 2–3 tablespoons (1 oz.) unfrosted whole grain breakfast cereal (less than 380 calories/100 g) and 6 pieces nuts (almonds, walnuts, cashews…).

- ¾ cup (6 oz.) plain nonfat yogurt, with sweetener if desired, *or* equivalent protein.

- 1 piece (5 oz.) fruit.

Mid-morning

- Black coffee, tea, or herbal tea in unlimited quantities, with sweetener and 2 tablespoons (1 fl. oz.) of skim milk, if desired.

Lunch

- Raw vegetables or salad in unlimited quantities seasoned with 1 teaspoon oil and unlimited lemon juice, vinegar, mustard, shallots, onion, herbs.

- 4 oz. lean meat, cooked without fat, *or* equivalent protein.

to diffuse, then strain. Whenever you boil vegetables for a meal, retain the water after cooking and refrigerate for later.

And remember, meat, fish, and vegetables must be cooked without fat. For extra flavor when cooking pasta or vegetables in water, you can use fat-free meat, chicken, or fish bouillon cubes. For salad dressings, do not use more than one teaspoon of oil or of light sour cream. Alternatively, you can allow yourself up to two tablespoons (1 oz.) of low-calorie commercial salad dressing (provided that you choose one that contains no more than 300 calories per 3 ½ oz.).

You can use as much sweetener as you like. Available in solid, powder, or liquid form, they are useful for satisfying a sweet tooth without the drawback of extra calories.

- Vegetables boiled or steamed without fat, in unlimited quantities.

- ¾ cup (6 oz.) plain nonfat yogurt with sweetener if desired *or* equivalent protein.

- 1 piece (5 oz.) fruit.

Afternoon

- Black coffee, tea, or herbal tea in unlimited quantities, with sweetener and 2 tablespoons (1 fl. oz.) of skim milk, if desired.

Dinner

- Raw vegetables or salad in unlimited quantities seasoned with 1 teaspoon oil and unlimited lemon juice, vinegar, mustard, shallots, onion, herbs, *or* vegetable soup (max. 100 calories and 3.5 g fat per serving).

- 4 oz. lean meat, cooked without fat, *or* equivalent protein.

- 3 ½ oz. carbohydrates (pasta, rice, couscous, potatoes) with 1 level teaspoon (¼ oz.) butter or margarine.

- 1 oz. cheese (less than 50% milk fat) *or* equivalent protein.

- Vegetables, boiled or steamed without fat, in unlimited quantities.

- 1 piece (5 oz.) fruit.

Basic Vinaigrette

Basic vinagrette:

2 tablespoons oil
1 tablespoon mustard
3 tablespoons water
Salt and pepper

Prep time: 5 min. / Ready in: 5 min.

Mix ingredients together in a screwtop jar and shake to emulsify.

Herb Vinaigrette

Optional ingredients to add to the basic vinagrette (see above):

Smoothly blended tomatoes or carrot juice or other vegetable juice
Fresh herbs of your choice
Scant ½ cup (3 oz.) plain nonfat yogurt or ⅓ cup (2 ½ oz.) 1% milk fat cottage cheese

Carrot–Lemon Dressing

2 tablespoons carrot juice
½ tablespoon mustard
2 tablespoons chopped tarragon
3 tablespoons lemon juice
1 tablespoon raspberry vinegar
2 tablespoons olive oil
Salt and pepper

Prep time: 5 min. / Ready in: 5 min.

Mix ingredients together in a screwtop jar and shake to emulsify.

GOURMET: CONDIMENTS

Tomato Citrus Vinaigrette

½ cup (4 fl. oz.) tomato juice
Juice of 1 grapefruit
1 clove garlic, crushed
Juice of 1 orange
1 tablespoon chopped chervil
Juice of 1 lemon
1 tablespoon chopped chives
1 shallot, chopped
1 tablespoon chopped parsley
1 tablespoon chopped tarragon
Zest of 1 lemon
2 teaspoons olive oil
Mustard, to taste
Salt and pepper

Prep time: 5 min. / Ready in: 5 min.

Mix ingredients together in a screwtop jar and shake to emulsify.

Vegetable Vinaigrette

½ cup (4 fl. oz.) tomato juice
3 tablespoons grapefruit juice and/or lemon juice
½ cup (4 fl. oz.) carrot juice
⅓ cup (3 fl. oz.) celery juice
2 tablespoons olive oil
Salt and pepper

Prep time: 5 min. / Ready in: 5 min.

Mix ingredients together in a screwtop jar and shake to emulsify.

Yogurt Dressing (Diet Mayonnaise)

1 cup (8 oz.) plain nonfat yogurt
1 tablespoon white vinegar
1 egg yolk
1 tablespoon mustard
1 tablespoon lemon juice
Seeds from 1 vanilla bean
Salt and pepper
3 egg whites

Prep time: 5 min. / Ready in: 5 min.

Mix together all ingredients except egg whites. Beat egg whites until stiff, fold into dressing.

Gribiche Dressing

Yogurt Dressing (see above)
1 hard-boiled egg white, chopped
2 pickles, chopped
1 tablespoon chopped parsley
1 tablespoon chopped tarragon
1 tablespoon chopped chervil

Prep time: 5 min. / Ready in: 5 min. (add 5 min. more to prepare Yogurt Dressing)

Mix ingredients together.

Tip: serve with asparagus, potatoes, roasted chicken, etc.

Ravigote Sauce

Yogurt Dressing (see above)
2 tablespoons capers
½ onion, chopped
1 tablespoon chopped parsley
1 tablespoon chopped chervil

Prep time: 5 min. / Ready in: 5 min. (add 5 minutes more to prepare Yogurt Dressing)

Mix ingredients together.

Tip: Serve with vegetables, seafood, meat, or poultry.

GOURMET: CONDIMENTS

Marinade for Fish or Shellfish

1 tablespoon chopped chives

1 shallot, chopped

1 tablespoon sherry vinegar and/or basil vinegar

½ tablespoon mustard and/or pinch of garlic

2 tablespoons olive oil

Salt and pepper

Prep time: 5 min. / Ready in: 5 min.

Mix ingredients together in a screwtop jar and shake to emulsify.

Tomato Sauce

1 onion, finely chopped

1 clove garlic, crushed

1 tablespoon olive oil

4 large tomatoes (approximately 1 ½ lb.), peeled and seeded

Salt and pepper

Prep time: 10 min. / Cook time: 20 min. / Ready in: 30 min.

Sauté the onion and garlic in the olive oil until transparent. Add the tomatoes, salt, and pepper. Simmer for 15 minutes then blend with a blender.

BREAKFAST

Toast

Cook time: 3 min. / Ready in: 3 min.

1 slice (1 oz.) French bread

2 teaspoons (⅓ oz.) regular butter

Toast bread, spread with butter, and serve.

Yogurt

¾ cup (6 oz.) plain nonfat yogurt

Fruit

1 orange

LUNCH

Beet Salad

Prep time: 10 min. / Ready in: 10 min.

Large handful salad greens (e.g., baby spinach, sliced chicory, iceberg)

2 small cooked beets, diced

1 medium hard-boiled egg, diced

1 tablespoon lemon juice or vinegar

1 tablespoon chopped parsley

Salt and pepper

Put salad greens in a bowl, add beets, add egg. In a separate bowl, mix lemon juice or vinegar, parsley, and seasoning into a dressing. Dress salad and serve.

Stuffed Veal

Prep time: 10 min. / Cook time: 30 min. / Ready in: 40 min.

1 ¼ cups (4 oz.) sliced mushrooms

1 slice (1 oz.) lean ham, diced

2 tablespoons chopped tarragon

Pinch of nutmeg

Salt and pepper

3 oz. veal cutlet

1 cup (8 fl. oz.) tomato juice

1 clove garlic, crushed

Preheat oven to 350°F. Chop ¼ cup of the mushrooms, mix with ham, tarragon, nutmeg, and salt and pepper. Make a slit lengthwise in the veal cutlet, and stuff with the vegetable mixture. Pour the tomato juice into a baking dish and place the veal on top. Roast for about 30 minutes. Meanwhile, sauté crushed garlic in a nonstick frying pan with remaining mushrooms and a little water. Season with salt and pepper and serve with the veal.

Fruit

1 apple

Grapefruit, Cottage Cheese, and Shrimp Salad

½ grapefruit

¼ cup (2 oz.) 1% milk fat cottage cheese

2 oz. shrimp

1 tablespoon capers

Pinch of paprika

Salt and pepper

Prep time: 10 min. / Ready in: 10 min.

Cut grapefruit in half. Remove the pulp with a grapefruit knife. Remove the pith and cut into large cubes. Mix the cottage cheese, shrimp, capers, and paprika in a bowl, and season with salt and pepper. Mix in grapefruit cubes. Scrape any remaining pith from one grapefruit half, and serve salad in grapefruit peel "bowl."

Roast Beef Salad

2 oz. lean roast beef , diced

2 pickles

Large handful salad greens

Prep time: 5 min. / Ready in: 5 min.

Combine ingredients and serve.

Yogurt

⅓ cup (3 oz.) plain nonfat yogurt

GOURMET: CLASSIC

BREAKFAST

Pancake and Berry Yogurt

1 pancake

1 tablespoon maple syrup

1 cup (8 oz.) berries (fresh or frozen)

¾ cup (6 oz.) plain nonfat yogurt

Prep time: 1 min. / Cook time: 2 min. / Ready in: 3 min.

Heat pancake, top with maple syrup. Mix berries into yogurt. Serve.

LUNCH

Cucumber with Fresh Mint

¾ cup (3 ½ oz./1 medium) cucumber, thinly sliced and seeded

⅓ cup (3 oz.) plain nonfat yogurt

2 tablespoons finely chopped mint leaves

1 teaspoon canola oil

Prep time: 5 min. / Ready in: 5 min.

Mix all ingredients and serve cold.

Beef Burger with Green Peppers

4 oz. ground lean beef

1 teaspoon tomato paste

⅓ cup (2 oz.) chopped onion

2 tablespoons chopped parsley

1 teaspoon olive oil

Salt and pepper

½ cup (1 medium) green bell pepper, cut into strips

Lettuce, to serve

Prep time: 10 min. / Cook time: 30 min. / Ready in: 40 min.

Preheat oven to 350°F. Mix the ground beef with the tomato paste, chopped onion, parsley, olive oil, and salt and pepper, and form into a patty. Place in a baking dish with pepper strips, cover with foil, bake for about 30 minutes or as desired. Serve on a bed of fresh lettuce, topped with the green pepper.

GOURMET: CLASSIC

Fruit

1 orange

Cheese

1 oz. hard cheese (American, cheddar, Parmesan)

Cottage Cheese Dip

Prep time: 5 min. / Ready in: 5 min.

½ cup (4 oz.) 1% milk fat cottage cheese
1 tablespoon chopped chives
1 clove garlic, crushed
Small bunch baby carrots

Mix cottage cheese with chives and garlic. Cut baby carrots into slices and dip.

Cod Spinach with Rice

Prep time: 10 min. / Cook time: 25 min. / Ready in: 35 min.

⅛ cup (¾ oz.) uncooked brown rice (for ½ cup cooked)
1 teaspoon olive oil
½ cup (4 fl. oz.) dry white wine
½ cup (3 oz.) crushed tomatoes
⅓ cup (2 oz.) chopped onion
2 cups (1 lb.) frozen spinach
4 oz. cod fillet
Salt and pepper
2 tablespoons (1 oz.) light sour cream

Preheat oven to 400°F.
Rinse rice. Add olive oil to saucepan and heat with rice for 3 minutes, then add ½ cup water and bring to a boil over high heat. Turn heat to low, stir, then cover tightly and cook for about 20 minutes (follow package instructions) or until water evaporates.
Cook the wine, tomatoes, and onions in a saucepan on low heat for 10 minutes. Defrost the spinach in a saucepan or microwave.
Place the spinach in a baking dish, place the fish on top, and cover with the sauce. Season with salt and pepper. Cook for about 15 minutes until the fish is cooked through. Top fish and vegetables with sour cream and serve with the rice.

Fruit

1 pear

GOURMET: CLASSIC

BREAKFAST

Oatmeal

¼ cup (1 oz.) dry oatmeal (for ½ cup cooked)

1 cup (8 fl. oz.) skim milk

6 nuts

Prep time: 3 min. / Ready in: 3 min.

Heat the oatmeal with the milk, garnish with nuts and serve.

Fruit

1 apple

LUNCH

Artichoke Salad

1 cup (6 oz.) artichoke hearts

2 tablespoons Gribiche Dressing (see page 172)

Prep time: 7 min. / Ready in: 7 min.

Toss the artichokes with the Gribiche dressing and serve.

Lamb Chops and Broccoli

4 oz. lean lamb chops

1 teaspoon oregano

⅓ cup (3 oz.) broccoli florets

Prep time: 5 min. / Cook time: 15 min. / Ready in: 20 min.

Sprinkle the lamb chops with oregano and grill or broil until center is opaque or as desired. Steam broccoli until tender. Serve.

Yogurt

¾ cup (6 oz.) plain nonfat yogurt

Fruit

1 small banana

Sauerkraut with Turkey and Peas

4 oz. lean turkey breast

½ cup (2 ½ oz.) green peas

½ cup (2 ½ oz.) sauerkraut

2 servings Yogurt Dressing
(see page 172)

Prep time: 5 min. / Cook time: 15 min. / Ready in: 20 min.

Grill, broil, or dry-fry the turkey breast for around 10 minutes or until opaque in center. Heat peas in microwave or on stovetop. Combine the sauerkraut with the yogurt dressing. Serve turkey with vegetable sides.

Pineapple Cottage Cheese

½ cup (4 oz.) 1% milk fat cottage cheese

1 cup (5 oz.) fresh pineapple chunks

Prep time: 3 min. / Ready in: 3 min.

Mix together, serve.

GOURMET: CLASSIC

BREAKFAST

Cheddar Toast

Prep time: 3 min. / Ready in: 3 min.

1 slice (1 oz.) whole grain bread
1 oz. cheddar cheese

Toast bread, top with cheddar, serve.

Milk

1 cup (8 fl. oz.) skim milk

Fruit

1 kiwi

LUNCH

Egg Mimosa

Prep time: 10 min. / Chill time: 5 min. / Ready in: 15 min.

1 medium hard-boiled egg
1 teaspoon canola oil
1 teaspoon chopped parsley
⅓ cup (3 oz.) plain nonfat yogurt
Salt and pepper
1 teaspoon lemon juice
Lettuce leaves, to serve

Cut the boiled egg lengthwise and remove the yolk. Mash egg yolk with canola oil, parsley, yogurt, and salt and pepper. When everything is well blended, pour the lemon juice inside the boiled egg white and top with yolk mixture. Serve chilled on a bed of salad.

Steak with Shallots and Green Beans

Prep time: 3 min. / Cook time: 15 min. / Ready in: 18 min.

½ cup (2 oz.) chopped shallots
Salt and pepper
4 oz. beef steak
1 cup (8 oz.) green beans
1 tablespoon chopped parsley

Heat the shallots in a nonstick frying pan with 4 tablespoons water until soft; add salt and pepper with beef. Dry-fry beef steak with the shallots for about 10 minutes or as desired. Meanwhile, steam the green beans with the parsley for 10 minutes or until tender. Serve.

Apple Yogurt

Prep time: 3 min. / Ready in: 3 min.

⅓ cup (3 oz.) plain nonfat yogurt
1 apple, chopped

Mix together, serve.

Chicken with Vegetables

1 cup (4 oz.) bean sprouts

½ cup (2 oz./1 medium) grated carrot

½ cup (3 oz.) canned corn kernels, drained

4 tablespoons Basic Vinaigrette (see page 170)

3 slices (3 oz.) lean chicken deli meat

Cheese

1 slice (1 oz.) Swiss or Emmental cheese

Fruit

1 small banana

Prep time: 10 min. / Ready in: 10 min.

Mix the bean sprouts, carrots, and corn kernels together with the vinaigrette and serve with the sliced chicken.

GOURMET: CLASSIC

BREAKFAST

Croissant and Kiwi with Milk

Prep time: 2 min. / Ready in: 2 min.

Peel kiwi, slice, and serve alongside croissant with a glass of milk.

LUNCH

Grilled Halibut with Zucchini and Cauliflower

1 cup (8 oz.) cauliflower florets
1 zucchini, sliced
1 tomato, diced
1 onion, chopped
1 tablespoon chopped parsley
1 clove garlic, crushed
1 teaspoon olive oil
1 teaspoon hot sauce
Salt and pepper
4 oz. halibut

Prep time: 5 min. / Cook time: 20 min. / Ready in: 25 min.

Heat grill to high.
Steam the cauliflower for about 10 minutes or until tender; remove and then steam zucchini until tender.
Meanwhile, in a nonstick frying pan, sauté tomato, onion, parsley, garlic, and olive oil over low heat for 5 minutes. Add hot sauce and salt and pepper; simmer for 10 minutes. Sear fish on a very hot grill for 3 minutes on each side.
Serve halibut topped with the sauce alongside the vegetable sides.

Strawberry–Lemon Yogurt

Juice of ½ lemon
¾ cup (6 oz.) plain nonfat yogurt
1 cup (8 oz.) fresh strawberries

Prep time: 5 min. / Ready in: 5 min.

Blend the lemon juice with the yogurt. Slice the strawberries, mix into yogurt, and serve.

DINNER

Fennel Casserole

1 bulb fennel, sliced
½ cup (3 oz.) chopped tomatoes
1 onion, chopped
2 cloves garlic, crushed
Salt and pepper

Prep time: 5 min. / Cook time: 30 min. / Ready in: 35 min.

Preheat oven to 350°F. Blanch fennel in salted boiling water for 10 minutes. Drain. Place fennel in casserole with tomatoes. Add onion, garlic, and salt and pepper, cover, and cook for 20 minutes. Serve.

GOURMET: CLASSIC

Baked Salmon

4 oz. fresh salmon steak
½ cup (3 oz.) chopped tomato
¼ onion, sliced
2 cloves garlic, crushed
Sprig of parsley
1 tablespoon snipped chives
1 bay leaf
1 teaspoon thyme leaves
1 teaspoon fennel seeds
Salt and pepper

Prep time: 5 min. / Cook time: 25 min. / Ready in: 30 min.

Preheat oven to 400°F. Place the salmon steak on a bed of tomatoes in a baking dish. Add the rest of the ingredients and bake in the oven for 25 minutes until the center of the fish is cooked. Serve.

Quinoa

¼ cup (1 ½ oz.) dry quinoa
1 teaspoon olive oil

Prep time: 10 min. / Cook time: 35 min. / Ready in: 45 min.

Rinse quinoa in large bowl, drain through fine mesh strainer, let sit 10 minutes in strainer to dry. Heat in dry nonstick frying pan for about 5 minutes. Boil ½ cup water, add quinoa and olive oil, and let cook for about 15 minutes or until water is fully absorbed. Let sit 10 minutes, fluff with fork, and serve.
Note: You can prepare ahead of time and keep refrigerated.

Cherry Tomato Cottage Cheese

7 cherry tomatoes
½ cup (4 oz.) 1% milk fat cottage cheese

Prep time: 3 min. / Ready in: 3 min.

Slice cherry tomatoes in half, mix into cottage cheese, and serve.

Pineapple Compote

½ cup (4 fl. oz.) water
1 teaspoon powdered sweetener
1 teaspoon vanilla extract
1 cup (5 oz.) pineapple chunks (fresh or canned in light syrup, drained)

Prep time: 5 min. / Cook time: 10 min. and 30 min. to cool / Ready in: 45 min.

In a saucepan, combine water, sweetener, and vanilla extract. When the mixture comes to a boil, add the pineapple chunks and leave on low heat, covered, for about 10 minutes. Chill in refrigerator and serve cold.

BREAKFAST

French Toast

Prep time: 3 min. / Ready in: 3 min.

1 slice frozen plain French toast

2 teaspoons (⅓ oz.) butter

Heat French toast, spread with butter, serve.

Yogurt

¾ cup (6 oz.) plain nonfat yogurt

Fruit

1 small pear, diced

Cinnamon

Sprinkle pear with cinnamon, serve.

LUNCH

Steak Tartare

Prep time: 10 min. / Ready in: 10 min.

4 oz. very fresh steak, chopped finely

1 egg yolk

½ teaspoon mustard

½ onion, finely chopped

1 tablespoon chopped parsley

1 teaspoon capers

½ teaspoon Worcestershire sauce

Salt and pepper

Mix all the ingredients together, and serve immediately.

Note: if you don't want to eat raw meat, form mixture into a patty, dry-fry in a nonstick frying pan, and serve.

Cauliflower, Potato, and Apple Salad

2 small potatoes
¾ cup (6 oz.) plain nonfat yogurt
1 teaspoon canola oil
2 tablespoons fresh herbs
Pinch of paprika
Salt and pepper
½ cup (4 oz.) cauliflower florets
1 carrot (4 oz.), peeled and grated
1 small apple, peeled, seeded,
   and cut into sticks
1 stalk celery, deveined and grated

Prep time: 15 min. / Cook time: 5 min. / Ready in: 20 min.

Cook potatoes in microwave for 5 minutes, then slice. In a bowl, prepare the sauce by blending yogurt, oil, herbs, paprika, salt and pepper. Add all the vegetables and mix well. Serve.

DINNER

Roast Beef with Garden Vegetables

4 oz. beef roast
Salt and pepper
1 carrot (4 oz.), peeled and sliced
   thinly
1 small leek, cut lengthwise and
   sliced thinly
2 sage leaves
Juice of 1 lemon
1 large tomato, cut in half
2 tablespoons finely chopped
   chives
1 tablespoon chopped parsley
1 teaspoon paprika

Prep time: 10 min. / Cook time: 25 min. / Ready in: 35 min.

Preheat oven to 450°F. Rinse beef under cold water, dry it, rub it with salt and pepper and place in a casserole dish. Pour 3 tablespoons of hot water over the meat and add the sliced carrot, sliced leek, and sage leaves. Bake, uncovered, for 12 minutes, basting the meat with lemon juice from time to time. Then add tomato and more lemon juice, and continue baking for an additional 4–8 minutes or as desired.

Remove from oven, place the roast on a warmed plate and arrange the vegetables around it. Garnish with chives and parsley. Deglaze casserole with a little water, season with salt, pepper, and paprika, and pour over meat. Serve.

Cheese

½ cup (4 oz.) 1% milk fat cottage
   cheese

Fruit

1 cup (8 oz.) canned fruit in light
   syrup, drained

BREAKFAST

Ricotta Bagel

½ whole grain bagel

¼ cup (2 oz.) part-skim ricotta cheese

Prep time: 3 min. / Ready in: 3 min.

Toast bagel, spread with ricotta, serve.

Milk

1 cup (8 fl. oz.) skim milk

Fruit

1 small apple

LUNCH

Celery Sticks

2 stalks celery

2 servings Yogurt Dressing (see page 172)

Serve.

Scrambled Eggs and Vegetable Medley

2 medium eggs

½ cup (4 oz.) 1% milk fat cottage cheese

1 tablespoon chopped chives

1 cup (approximately 3 oz.) mixed vegetables, chopped

Prep time: 5 min. / Cook time: 5 min. / Ready in: 10 min.

Whisk eggs, then pour into pan and scramble with the cottage cheese and chives. Steam the vegetables and serve together.

Fruit

1 cup (4 oz.) grapes

GOURMET: CLASSIC

Steamed Tilapia with Basil

4 oz. tilapia (or other fish)

5 leaves basil, chopped

Prep time: 2 min. / Cook time: 13 min. / Ready in: 15 min.

Boil water and steam tilapia with basil for about 8 minutes or until center is opaque. Serve.

Pumpkin Gratin

1 cup (6 ½ oz.) pumpkin, chopped

¼ cup (2 fl. oz.) fat-free vegetable broth

1 egg yolk

Salt and pepper

¼ cup (1 oz.) grated cheese

Prep time: 5 min. / Cook time: 25 min. / Ready in: 30 min.

Boil or steam pumpkin until tender and drain well. Place pieces in a baking dish. Whisk together broth, egg yolk, and salt and pepper. Pour over the pumpkin and sprinkle with cheese. Broil until lightly golden. Serve.

Fruit

1 small orange

BREAKFAST

Toasted PB&J

1 slice (1 oz.) whole grain bread,
toasted

2 teaspoons peanut butter

2 teaspoons jam

Prep time: 3 min. / Ready in: 3 min.

Spread peanut butter and jam on toast.
Serve.

Yogurt

¾ cup (6 oz.) plain nonfat yogurt

LUNCH

Tuna Salad

1 can tuna packed in water,
drained

1 cup (4 oz.) reduced-fat cheese,
diced

2 stalks celery, diced

1 medium hard-boiled egg, diced

2 tablespoons capers

Pinch of chili powder

1 bell pepper, diced

1 onion, minced

1 tablespoon lemon juice

1 teaspoon canola oil

1 teaspoon hot sauce

1 handful lettuce, shredded

½ cup (2 oz./1 small) cucumber,
sliced

Prep time: 10 min. / Ready in: 10 min.

Put the tuna in a bowl and separate with a
fork. Mix in cheese, celery, hard-boiled egg,
capers, chili, pepper, onion, lemon juice, oil,
and hot sauce. Serve on a bed of lettuce and
garnish with cucumber slices.

Fruit

1 pear

Veal Cutlet with Oven-baked Carrots

1 cup (8 oz.) diced carrots

¼ cup (2 oz.) chopped onion

2 tablespoons chopped parsley

½ teaspoon curry powder

1 teaspoon olive oil

3 oz. veal cutlet

1 teaspoon chopped rosemary

Salt and pepper

2 tablespoons (1 oz.) light sour cream

Prep time: 5 min. / Cook time: 45 min. / Ready in: 50 min.

Preheat oven to 375°F. Mix carrots, onion, parsley, curry powder, and olive oil in a baking dish. Cover with aluminum foil and roast for 45 minutes. Meanwhile, season the veal with rosemary and salt and pepper, and grill or broil for about 10–15 minutes or as desired. Serve with sour cream.

Polenta

½ cup (2 oz.) polenta (cornmeal)

Salt and pepper

Prep time: 4 min. / Cook time: 10 min. / Ready in: 14 min.

Boil 2 cups water, add polenta. Simmer on low heat, stirring for around 10 minutes (see package instructions) until polenta softens. Add salt and pepper to taste, serve.

Cheese

1 oz. hard cheese (American, cheddar, Parmesan)

Fruit

1 small apple

GOURMET: CLASSIC

BREAKFAST

Cereal

2–3 tablespoons (1 oz.) unfrosted whole grain cereal

1 cup (8 fl. oz.) skim milk

Prep time: 2 min. / Ready in: 2 min.

Pour cereal and milk into bowl, serve.

Nuts

6 almonds

Fruit

1 small banana

LUNCH

Poached Salmon

4 oz. salmon

Prep time: 1 min. / Cook time: 10 min. / Ready in: 11 min.

Place salmon, skin-side down, in a non-stick frying pan, add water just to the top of the salmon. Cook over high heat for 4 minutes. Turn the salmon over and then continue cooking for an additional 5–6 minutes. Serve.

Garden Salad

1 cup (2 oz.) shredded lettuce

1 (2 oz.) tomato, sliced

½ cup (2 oz./1 small) cucumber, sliced

¼ cup sliced celery

3 ears baby corn

Juice of 1 lemon

1 tablespoon Ravigote Dressing (see page 172)

Prep time: 10 min. / Ready in: 10 min.

Mix vegetables in a bowl, drizzle with lemon juice, and toss with the ravigote dressing. Serve.

Cheese

½ cup (4 oz.) 1% milk fat cottage cheese

Fruit

1 (4 oz.) peach

Sirloin Steak with Italian-style Eggplant

Cooking spray
1 cup (3 oz.) sliced eggplant
1 cup (3 ¼ oz.) diced mushrooms
1 tablespoon chopped onion
Salt and pepper
1 tablespoon chopped parsley
4 oz. sirloin steak

Prep time: 20 min. / Cook time: 25 min. / Ready in: 45 min.

Place eggplant in salted water for 20 minutes then drain, rinse, and dry. Coat nonstick frying pan with cooking spray, fry eggplant for 5 minutes until golden brown. Add mushrooms, onion, a few tablespoons water, and salt and pepper. Cover and cook on a low heat for 15 minutes. Add parsley and cook 5 minutes more. Meanwhile, grill or broil the steak for 5 minutes. Serve.

Pasta

¼ cup (1 oz.) dry pasta (for ½ cup cooked)
1 teaspoon butter

Prep time: 4 min. / Cook time: 8 min. / Ready in: 12 min.

Boil water, add pasta and cook according to package instructions. Drain, return to saucepan and add butter, mix and serve.

Yogurt

¾ cup (6 oz.) plain nonfat yogurt

Fruit

1 slice (5 oz.) mango

GOURMET: CLASSIC

BREAKFAST

Bagel and Scrambled Egg

½ whole grain bagel
1 medium egg
¼ cup (2 oz.) part-skim ricotta cheese

Prep time: 3 min. / Cook time: 7 min. / Ready in: 10 min.

Toast bagel. In the meantime, whisk egg, cook over medium heat in dry, nonstick saucepan. Spread ricotta cheese on bagel. Serve.

Berry Smoothie

1 cup (8 oz.) frozen berries

Prep time: 4 min. / Ready in: 4 min.

Liquify berries in a blender, adding water if desired, and serve.

LUNCH

Light Sauerkraut

1 can (5 oz.) natural sauerkraut, drained
4 oz. pork tenderloin
1 small apple, peeled, cored, and sliced thickly
Salt and pepper
1 slice (1 oz.) smoked ham, diced

Prep time: 5 min. / Cook time: 30 min. / Ready in: 35 min.

Preheat oven to 350°F. Place half of the sauerkraut in a casserole, add the tenderloin and apple slices. Season wih salt and pepper. Top with remaining sauerkraut, and cover. Bake for 20 minutes, add ham, and cook for an additional 10 minutes. Serve.

Yogurt

¾ cup (6 oz.) plain nonfat yogurt

Corn Salad

2 tablespoons Basic Vinaigrette (see page 170)

½ cup canned corn kernels

Prep time: 7 min. / Ready in: 7 min.

Prepare vinaigrette, toss with corn, and serve.

Baked Leeks

2 leeks

1 medium egg, beaten

½ cup (4 fl. oz.) skim milk

½ cup (2 oz.) finely chopped lean ham

Salt and pepper

Prep time: 5 min. / Cook time: 1 hour / Ready in: 1 hour 5 min.

Preheat oven to 350°F. Cut leeks into slices ½ inch thick and place in a baking dish. Beat the egg with milk and pour mixture over the leeks. Add ham and salt and pepper. Cover the dish with foil and bake for about 1 hour. Uncover and serve.

Cheese

¼ cup (2 oz.) 1% milk fat cottage cheese

Fruit

1 small pear

BREAKFAST

Oatmeal

⅓ cup (1 oz.) dry oats
1 cup (8 fl. oz.) skim milk

Cook time: 7 min. / Ready in: 7 min.

Heat oats and milk in a saucepan for 5 minutes and let sit for 2 minutes (or follow package instructions). Serve.

Nuts

6 nuts

Fruit

2 tablespoons raisins

LUNCH

Radishes

1 cup (about 12) chopped radishes
2 tablespoons Herb Vinaigrette (see page 170)

Prep time: 5 min. / Ready in: 5 min.

Top radishes with vinaigrette and serve.

Stuffed Tomatoes

3 oz. lean ground beef
1 medium egg, beaten
2 tablespoons chopped mixed herbs
Salt and pepper
2 large tomatoes

Prep time: 5 min. / Cook time: 35 min. / Ready in: 40 min.

Preheat oven to 400°F. Mix ground beef, egg, herbs, and salt and pepper to make a stuffing. Core the tomatoes, fill with the stuffing, and bake for 35 minutes. Serve.

Cheese

½ cup (4 oz.) 1% milk fat cottage cheese

Fruit

1 pear

Coleslaw

1 cup (3 oz.) shredded vegetable
coleslaw

2 tablespoons Yogurt Dressing
(see page 172)

Prep time: 3 min. / Ready in: 3 min.

Toss the coleslaw in the dressing and serve.

Baked Pollock
with Herb Cream

4 oz. pollock fillet

Salt and pepper

¼ cup (2 oz.) 1% milk fat cottage
cheese

1 clove garlic, crushed

1 tablespoon chopped parsley

½ tablespoon lemon juice

Prep time: 5 min. / Cook time: 20 min. / Ready in: 25 min.

Preheat oven to 375°F. Season pollock fillet
with salt and pepper and set aside. Mix
cottage cheese, garlic, parsley, and salt and
pepper. Spread the mixture on the pollock
fillet. Bake in a baking dish for 20 minutes.
Drizzle with lemon juice and serve.

Spinach

1 cup (1 oz.) spinach

2 tablespoons (1 oz.) light sour
cream

Prep time: 4 min. / Ready in: 4 min.

Sauté spinach in a dry nonstick pan,
mix in sour cream. Serve.

Pasta

¼ cup dry pasta (for ½ cup
cooked)

Boil pasta in salted water per package
instructions, serve.

Fruit

4 apricots

GOURMET: CLASSIC

BREAKFAST

Melba Toast

2 teaspoons (⅓ oz.) butter
2 tablespoons fruit jam
4 slices melba toast

Prep time: 2 min. / Ready in: 2 min.

Spread butter and jam on melba toast, serve.

Milk

1 cup (8 fl. oz.) skim milk

LUNCH

Vegetable

8 baby carrots

Baked Lamb

4 oz. extra-lean lamb leg
1 clove garlic, crushed
½ cup chopped parsley
1 tablespoon dried rosemary
Salt and pepper
½ cup (4 fl. oz.) fat-free beef broth
1 small red chili pepper, marinated in water or vinegar

Prep time: 5 min. / Cook time: 20 min. / Ready in: 25 min.

Preheat oven to 350°F. Remove all visible fat from the lamb. Rub the meat with garlic and herbs. Sprinkle with salt and pepper. Place the lamb in a baking pan with the beef broth, bake for 20 minutes. Slice the red chili into thin pieces and sprinkle over the meat. Serve.

Green Beans with Capers

1 cup (5 ½ oz.) green beans
1 tomato, chopped
1 clove garlic, crushed
1 tablespoon chopped tarragon
1 teaspoon capers
½ lemon, sliced
Salt and pepper

Prep time: 5 min. / Cook time: 15 min. / Ready in: 20 min.

Blanch beans in salted boiling water. Heat the tomato and crushed garlic in a nonstick saucepan. Add the green beans and cook on very low heat for 10 minutes. Add tarragon and capers 5 minutes before serving. Garnish with lemon slices, season with salt and pepper. Serve.

Cheese

¼ cup (2 oz.) part-skim ricotta
cheese

Fruit

½ grapefruit

DINNER

Salad

Several leaves iceberg lettuce,
shredded

4 tablespoons Basic Vinaigrette
(see page 170)

Prep time: 2 min. / Ready in: 2 min.

Dress lettuce with vinaigrette and serve.

Zucchini Lasagne

1 (5 oz.) zucchini, cut into strips
lengthwise

¼ cup (2 oz.) onion, chopped

2 tablespoons Tomato Sauce
(see page 173)

4 oz. tuna packed in brine,
drained

1 tablespoon chopped basil

Salt and pepper

¼ cup (2 oz.) grated reduced-fat
cheddar cheese

Prep time: 10 min. / Cook time: 30 min. / Ready in: 40 min.

Blanch zucchini for 2–3 minutes in salted
boiling water (or microwave). Dry-fry onion
in a dry nonstick pan. Add tomato sauce,
along with drained flaked tuna, basil,
and salt and pepper. Layer a baking dish
with the strips of zucchini and the tomato
sauce. Top with grated cheese and bake for
25 minutes. Serve.

Rice

⅛ cup (¾ oz.) uncooked brown
rice (for ½ cup cooked)

1 teaspoon olive oil

Prep time: 5 min. / Cook time: 20 min. / Ready in: 25 min.

Rinse rice. Add olive oil to saucepan and
heat with rice for 3 minutes, then add ½ cup
water and bring to a boil over high heat.
Turn heat to low, stir, then cover tightly and
cook for about 20 minutes (follow package
instructions) or until water evaporates.

Fruit

½ cup mixed fruit compote
with no added sugar

GOURMET: CLASSIC

BREAKFAST

Cereal

Prep time: 2 min. / Ready in: 2 min.

2–3 tablespoons (1 oz.) unfrosted whole grain cereal

1 cup (8 fl. oz.) skim milk

Pour cereal and milk into bowl, serve.

Nuts

6 walnuts

Fruit

1 small orange

LUNCH

Carrot–Chive Salad

Prep time: 3 min. / Ready in: 3 min.

1 cup (2 medium) grated carrots

1 tablespoon chopped chives

2 tablespoons Basic Vinaigrette (see page 170)

Toss ingredients together, serve.

Steak with Garlic Butter

Prep time: 5 min. / Cook time: 10 min. / Ready in: 15 min.

1 teaspoon (¼ oz.) butter

1 tablespoon chopped parsley

½ garlic clove, crushed

Salt and pepper

4 oz. lean sirloin steak

Mix butter, parsley, garlic, and season with salt and pepper. In a nonstick frying pan, dry-fry the steak for a few minutes on both sides without fat. Serve steak with pat of garlic butter on top.

Baked Eggplant

Prep time: 30 min. / Cook time: 45 min. / Ready in: 1 hour 15 min.

1 large (4 oz.) eggplant

1 clove garlic, crushed

1 onion, chopped

½ cup (3 oz.) chopped fennel

1 tablespoon chopped parsley

Preheat oven to 400°F. Peel eggplant and cut into slices ½ inch thick. Place in salted water for 20 minutes then drain, rinse, and dry. Place in a baking dish and top with the

GOURMET: CLASSIC

⅓ cup (3 fl. oz.) tomato juice
¼ cup (1 oz.) grated cheese
Salt and pepper

vegetables and parsley, cover with tomato juice, and sprinkle with cheese. Cook for 45 minutes. Serve.

Fruit

1 cup (8 oz.) fruit in light syrup, drained

DINNER

Vegetable Soup

1 cup fat-free vegetable soup (less than 100 calories per serving)

Cook time: 5 min. / Ready in: 5 min.

Heat and serve.

Lemon Chicken and Mushrooms

4 oz. chicken breast
Zest of 1 lemon
Salt and pepper
1 cup (3 ¼ oz.) sliced mushrooms
1 clove garlic, crushed
1 tablespoon chopped parsley

Prep time: 5 min. / Cook time: 30 min. / Ready in: 35 min.

Preheat oven to 350°F. Place chicken in a baking dish and sprinkle with lemon zest and salt and pepper. Bake for 30 minutes. Meanwhile, sauté the mushrooms with garlic and parsley in a dry nonstick frying pan. Serve.

Semolina

⅓ cup dry semolina (for ½ cup cooked semolina)

Prep time: 4 min. / Cook time: 4 min. / Ready in: 8 min.

Heat 1 ½ cups water in a saucepan. When water begins to simmer, stir in semolina, and continue stirring for 2 minutes (follow package instructions) until water evaporates. Serve.

Yogurt

¾ cup (6 oz.) plain nonfat yogurt

Fruit

1 cup (5 oz.) fresh pineapple chunks

BREAKFAST

Whole Grain Toast

1 slice (1 oz.) whole grain bread
2 teaspoons (⅓ oz.) regular
  butter

Prep time: 3 min. / Ready in: 3 min.

Toast the bread, keep warm, spread with butter. Serve.

Yogurt

¾ cup (6 oz.) plain nonfat yogurt

Juice

1 cup (8 fl. oz.) fresh orange juice

LUNCH

Spinach Salad

4 oz. crab sticks, cut into slices
2 cups (2 oz.) fresh spinach
½ cup (4 oz.) 1% milk fat cottage
  cheese
½ cup (1 ½ oz.) sliced
  mushrooms
1 shallot, chopped
1 tomato, chopped
1 clove garlic, crushed
Salt and pepper
1 serving Tomato Citrus
  Vinaigrette (see page 171)

Prep time: 5 min. / Ready in: 5 min.

Mix all ingredients in a bowl, toss with vinaigrette. Serve.

Fruit

½ grapefruit

Artichoke Salad

Prep time: 3 min. / Cook time: 35 min. / Ready in: 38 min.

1 artichoke

2 tablespoons Yogurt Dressing
(see page 172)

Trim artichoke stem and steam for
35 minutes or until tender. Serve with
side of dressing for dipping.

Baked Ham

Prep time: 10 min. / Cook time: 25 min. / Ready in: 35 min.

1 (3 oz.) carrot

1 (3 oz.) turnip

1 cup (3 oz.) green beans

1 stalk celery

Salt and pepper

4 oz. (thick slice) ham

¼ cup (2 fl. oz.) white wine

Preheat oven to 350°F. Cut vegetables into
thin julienne strips. Mix and season with
salt and pepper. Place half the vegetables in
a baking dish and add the ham. Cover with
the remaining vegetables, pour over the
wine, and cover. Bake for 25 minutes. Serve.

Mashed Potatoes

Prep time: 3 min. / Cook time: 15 min. / Ready in: 18 min.

1 medium (4 oz.) potato, peeled
and diced

2 tablespoons (1 oz.) light sour
cream

Boil or microwave 1 medium potato until
tender. Mash. Mix ½ cup mashed potatoes
with sour cream. Serve.

Yogurt

¾ cup (6 oz.) plain nonfat yogurt

Fruit

1 small apple

BREAKFAST

Toast

1 slice (1 oz.) French bread
1 teaspoon (¼ oz.) regular butter

Prep time: 5 min. / Ready in: 5 min.

Toast bread, spread with butter, and serve.

Yogurt

¾ cup (6 oz.) plain nonfat yogurt

Fruit

1 kiwi

LUNCH

Shrimp Salad with Beets and Corn

½ cup (2 oz.) baby corn
½ cup (2 oz.) diced beets
1 tablespoon vinegar
4 oz. shrimp

Prep time: 5 min. / Ready in: 5 min.

Combine all ingredients and serve.

Yogurt

¾ cup (6 oz.) plain nonfat yogurt

Fruit

1 apple

Carpaccio with Potato Salad

Prep time: 10 min. / Cook time: 25 min. and 30 min. to cool / Ready in: 65 min.

1 medium (4 oz.) potato
Sea salt and pepper
2 tablespoons olive oil
1 oz. Parmesan cheese
4 oz. beef carpaccio, thinly sliced
6 basil leaves

Place potato in a pot of cold salted water. Cook for about 25 minutes. Drain, peel, and cut into ⅛-inch slices. Place in a bowl with half the olive oil. Season with salt and pepper and set aside for 30 minutes to cool. Shave the Parmesean into curls.
Pour remaining oil into a shallow dish and dip the slices of meat in it.
Place the potatoes on a plate, arrange the meat on top, and add the Parmesan cheese and basil. Add a pinch of salt and pepper. Serve.

Salad

Prep time: 2 min. / Ready in 2 min.

Several leaves iceberg lettuce
1 tablespoon balsamic vinegar

Toss lettuce in balsamic vinegar and serve.

Fruit

1 slice (5 oz.) mango

GOURMET: POTATO

BREAKFAST

Bagel

½ whole grain bagel

Prep time: 5 min. / Ready in: 5 min.

Toast bagel, serve.

Milk

1 cup (8 fl. oz.) skim milk

Cheese

⅓ cup (3 oz.) 1% milk fat cottage cheese

Fruit

1 small pear

LUNCH

Chicken Salad with Grated Carrots

4 oz. cooked chicken breast, diced
1 cup (6 oz./2 large) grated carrots
1 tablespoon chopped chives
Juice of ½ lemon
Salt and pepper

Prep time: 10 min. / Ready in: 10 min.

Combine ingredients and serve.

Baked Eggplant

1 large (4 oz.) eggplant
1 clove garlic, crushed
1 onion, chopped
½ cup (3 oz.) chopped fennel
1 tablespoon chopped parsley
⅓ cup (3 fl. oz.) tomato juice
¼ cup (1 oz.) grated cheese
Salt and pepper

Prep time: 30 min. / Cook time: 45 min. / Ready in: 1 hour 15 min.

Preheat oven to 400°F. Peel eggplant and cut into slices ½ inch thick. Place in salted water for 20 minutes then drain, rinse, and dry. Place in a baking dish and top with the vegetables and parsley, cover with tomato juice, and sprinkle with cheese. Cook for 45 minutes. Serve.

Strawberry Yogurt

Prep time: 3 min. / Ready in: 3 min.

¾ cup (6 oz.) fresh strawberries, sliced

¾ cup (6 oz.) plain nonfat yogurt

Mix strawberries into yogurt and serve.

DINNER

Potato Salad with Artichoke Hearts, Feta, and Lemon

4 oz. Russet potatoes

¼ oz. (about 30) pine nuts

¼ preserved lemon (1 oz.)

1 cup (7 oz.) canned artichoke hearts

1 tablespoon olive oil

½ onion, minced

½ bunch cilantro, minced

Salt and pepper

1 small orange

Juice of 1 lemon

¼ cup (2 oz.) crumbled reduced-fat feta cheese

Prep time: 10 min. / Cook time: 25 min. / Ready in: 35 min.

Place potatoes in a pot of cold salted water, cook over high heat for 25 minutes. Meanwhile, dry roast the pine nuts in a nonstick frying pan. Rinse and chop preserved lemon. Cut artichoke hearts into quarters. Drain the potato, peel, and cut into small cubes. Pour into a bowl and drizzle with olive oil. Stir in artichoke quarters, lemon, onion, and cilantro. Add salt and pepper and mix.

Meanwhile, using a vegetable peeler, remove the zest from the orange, cut into sections and blanch in boiling water for about 30 seconds. Add to salad with the pine nuts. Drizzle with lemon juice and toss. Sprinkle the feta over the salad and serve.

Ham

3 slices (3 oz.) lean ham

Fruit

1 medium peach

GOURMET: POTATO

BREAKFAST

Hot Chocolate

1 cup (8 fl. oz.) hot skim milk

2 tablespoons powdered hot chocolate mix

Prep time: 2 min. / Cook time: 5 min. / Ready in: 7 min.

Put powdered chocolate mix in mug, add milk and stir. Microwave for 3–5 minutes or until hot. Stir and serve.

Pastry

1 small (2 ½ oz.) sweet roll (less than 150 kcal per serving)

LUNCH

Leeks

2 leeks, sliced lengthwise

2 tablespoons Basic Vinaigrette (see page 170)

Prep time: 5 min. / Cook time: 8 min. / Ready in: 13 min.

Steam leeks for about 8 minutes or until tender. Dress with vinaigrette and serve.

Steamed Cod and Cauliflower

4 oz. cod fillet

1 tablespoon chopped basil

½ cup (4 oz.) cauliflower florets

Prep time: 5 min. / Cook time: 15 min. / Ready in: 20 min.

Steam the cod with the basil for 5 minutes or until opaque in center. Boil or steam the cauliflower for 10 minutes or until tender. Serve.

Yogurt

¾ cup (6 oz.) plain nonfat yogurt

Fruit

1 small orange

GOURMET: POTATO

Mackerel Potato Salad

4 oz. Russet potatoes

4 oz. smoked mackerel fillet

½ cup (4 oz.) 1% milk fat cottage cheese

1 small onion, minced

1 tablespoon chopped chives

Salt and pepper

1 tablespoon olive oil

1 tablespoon white wine vinegar

1 handful shredded lettuce

Prep time: 10 min. / Cook time: 25 min. / Ready in: 35 min.

Place potatoes in a pot of cold salted water, cook for about 25 minutes. Drain the potatoes, let cool, peel and cut into thick slices. Remove skin and any bones from mackerel, and mix together in a bowl, with the cottage cheese, onion, and chives. Lightly season with salt and pepper. Prepare vinaigrette with olive oil, vinegar, and salt and pepper. In a bowl, gently toss all ingredients together. Serve.

Fruit

2 plums

BREAKFAST

Cereal

2–3 tablespoons (1 oz.) unfrosted whole grain cereal

1 cup (8 fl. oz.) skim milk

Prep time: 2 min. / Ready in: 2 min.

Pour cereal and milk into bowl, serve.

Milk

1 cup (8 fl. oz.) skim milk

Nuts

6 almonds

Fruit

1 kiwi

LUNCH

Salad

Handful shredded lettuce

2 tablespoons Yogurt Dressing (see page 172)

Prep time: 2 min. / Ready in: 2 min.

Toss lettuce with yogurt dressing and serve.

Omelet

2 medium eggs

Prep time: 2 min. / Cook time 8 min. / Ready in: 10 min.

Whisk eggs, heat in a dry nonstick frying pan over medium heat, stirring frequently. Serve.

Broccoli

1 cup (4 oz.) broccoli

Prep time: 2 min. / Cook time 10 min. / Ready in: 12 min.

Steam broccoli for 10 minutes or until tender. Serve.

Yogurt

¾ cup (6 oz.) plain nonfat yogurt

Fruit

½ grapefruit

Potato and Scallop Medley

4 oz. yellow potatoes

1 medium egg

2 oz. scallops

1 stalk celery, grated

¼ cup (2 oz.) sliced onion

½ cup (4 oz.) 1% milk fat cottage cheese

½ teaspoon mustard

Juice of ½ lemon

1 tablespoon canola oil

3 sprigs parsley, chopped

3 sprigs chives, chopped

1 sprig mint, chopped

Salt and pepper

Sorbet

2 scoops (2 oz.) of sorbet

Prep time: 15 min. / Cook time: 30 min. and 15 min. to chill / Ready in: 60 min.

Place potatoes in a pot of cold salted water; bring to a boil and cook for about 25 minutes. Drain the potatoes, let cool. Cook the egg for 5 minutes in boiling water and rinse under cool water.

Meanwhile, sauté scallops in a nonstick frying pan for about 5 minutes or until opaque in center. Chop half and reserve the remaining half for dressing the dish. Peel the potatoes and cut 2 tablespoons of potato flesh into small cubes. In a bowl, toss scallops, egg, celery, onions, and cubed potato. In another bowl, mix cottage cheese with mustard, lemon juice, canola oil, and the herbs. Season with salt and pepper. Pour the dressing over the potato mixture, mix, and arrange on plate or in a decorative scallop shell. Garnish with the remaining scallops. Serve chilled.

GOURMET: POTATO

Breakfast

Cheese and Crackers

2 reduced-fat crispbread crackers
(about 1 oz.)
1 slice (1 oz.) cheddar cheese

Prep time: 2 min. / Ready in: 2 min.

Top crackers with cheese and serve.

Yogurt

¾ cup (6 oz.) plain nonfat yogurt

Fruit Juice

1 cup (8 fl. oz.) freshly squeezed
orange juice

Lunch

Avocado

½ avocado, diced
1 tablespoon lemon juice

Prep time: 2 min. / Ready in: 2 min.

Dress avocado with lemon juice, serve.

Salmon with Zucchini

4 oz. salmon fillet
1 tablespoon chopped dill
2 medium zucchini, sliced
1 teaspoon olive oil

Prep time: 10 min. / Cook time: 15 min. / Ready in: 25 min.

Grill or broil the salmon fillet for about
5 minutes or until center is opaque.
Season with the dill. Cook the zucchini
in a nonstick frying pan with the olive oil
for about 10 minutes. Serve.

Yogurt

¾ cup (6 oz.) plain nonfat yogurt

Stuffed Potatoes

4 oz. yellow potatoes
1 tablespoon olive oil
1 onion, chopped
1 shallot, chopped
3 oz. lean ham, diced finely
½ cup (1 ¼ oz.) shiitake
  mushrooms, diced finely
Salt and pepper

Cheese

½ cup (4 oz.) 1% milk fat cottage
  cheese

Fruit

1 cup (5 oz.) fresh pineapple
  chunks

Prep time: 10 min. / Cook time: 35 min. / Ready in: 45 min.

Place the potatoes in a pot of cold salted water. Bring to a boil and cook for about 25 minutes. Drain the potatoes, let them cool. Cut the potatoes in two lengthwise and scoop the flesh out. Heat oil in a nonstick frying pan, add onion and shallot and stir until browned. Add ham and mushrooms and cook for 4 minutes, stirring occasionally. Add potato flesh and mix with salt and pepper.

Fill the potato skins with the stuffing. Arrange in a baking dish with a little water. Cook for 5 minutes under broiler. Serve.

GOURMET: POTATO

BREAKFAST

Cheese and Crackers

2 reduced-fat crispbread crackers
(about 1 oz.)
2 tablespoons (1 oz.) part-skim
ricotta cheese

Prep time: 2 min. / Ready in: 2 min.

Top crackers with cheese and serve.

Milk

1 cup (8 fl. oz.) skim milk

Fruit

¾ (3 oz.) cup grapes

LUNCH

Bean Sprout Salad

⅝ cup (2 ½ oz.) bean sprouts
2 sprigs cilantro, chopped
2 tablespoons Basic Vinaigrette
(see page 170)

Prep time: 2 min. / Ready in: 2 min.

Dress bean sprouts and cilantro with
vinaigrette and serve.

Grilled Chicken with Chinese Vegetables

4 oz. chicken breast
½ tablespoon soy sauce
1 cup (5 oz.) frozen stir-fried
Chinese vegetables

Prep time: 5 min. / Cook time: 15 min. / Ready in: 20 min.

Season chicken with soy sauce and grill
or broil for 10 minutes or until opaque in
center. Heat vegetables. Serve.

Fruit

¾ cup (6 oz.) fruit in light syrup,
drained

Potato Pancake (Rösti) with Smoked Haddock

Prep time: 10 min. / Cook time: 30 min. / Ready in: 40 min.

1 cup (8 fl. oz.) water

½ cup (4 fl. oz.) skim milk

4 oz. smoked haddock fillet

4 oz. white potatoes, peeled

1 onion, finely chopped

Salt and pepper

1 teaspoon oil

2 tablespoons (1 oz.) light sour cream

1 shallot, minced

6 sprigs parsley, chopped

Heat the water and milk in a pot. Add the fish and poach for 10 minutes. Drain and set aside. Grate potatoes coarsely into a bowl; add onion and salt lightly. Warm oil in a nonstick frying pan. Add the potatoes and shape into a thick slab using a wooden spoon. Cook for 10 minutes until a crust forms. Using a lid or plate to help, flip the pancake and cook for another 10 minutes. Flake the haddock into a bowl. Add sour cream and shallots and toss gently. Serve over potato pancake, sprinkled with chopped parsley.

Yogurt

¾ cup (6 oz.) plain nonfat yogurt

Fruit

1 cup (6 oz.) frozen berries

GOURMET: POTATO

BREAKFAST

Egg and Toast

1 slice (1 oz.) whole grain bread
1 medium hard-boiled egg

Prep time: 3 min. / Ready in: 3 min.

Toast bread, serve with egg.

Cheese

½ cup (4 oz.) 1% milk fat cottage
cheese

LUNCH

Tomato Salad

1 cup (6 oz.) diced tomatoes
2 tablespoons Basic Vinaigrette
(see page 170)

Prep time: 3 min. / Ready in: 3 min.

Toss and serve.

Beef Burger
with Vegetables

4 oz. ground lean beef
4 oz. frozen vegetables
1 teaspoon Dijon mustard

Prep time: 5 min. / Cook time: 10 min. / Ready in: 15 min.

Grill or dry-fry the burger for about
10 minutes or as desired. Heat the
vegetables in a saucepan or microwave.
Serve with mustard.

Yogurt

¾ cup (6 oz.) plain nonfat yogurt

Fruit

1 cup (6 oz.) fresh berries

Mashed Potato Tartar

4 oz. white potatoes, peeled and cut into large cubes

¼ cup (2 fl. oz.) skim milk

2 teaspoons (⅓ oz.) butter

4 oz. tuna packed in water, drained

½ cup (2 oz.) pickles

Sprig of dill, chopped

1 tablespoon mustard

Salt and white pepper

Prep time: 5 min. / Cook time: 25 min. / Ready in: 30 min.

Steam potatoes for 25 minutes or until tender. Bring milk to a boil. Add potatoes and butter to milk; mash. Drain tuna and flake. Drain and slice pickles. Mix potatoes with tuna, pickles, dill, mustard, salt and pepper. Serve.

Yogurt

¾ cup (6 oz.) plain nonfat yogurt

Fruit

1 apple

BREAKFAST

Yogurt

¾ cup (6 oz.) plain nonfat yogurt

Fruit

¾ cup (6 oz.) fruit in light syrup,
   drained

LUNCH

Cucumber and Tomato Salad

½ cup (2 oz./1 small) cucumber,
   sliced
1 medium tomato, diced
1 serving Basic Vinaigrette (see
   page 170)

Prep time: 5 min. / Ready in: 5 min.

Toss cucumber and tomato in vinaigrette, and serve.

Sardine and Fennel Linguine

1 tablespoon olive oil
½ onion, chopped
1 clove garlic, unpeeled
1 bulb fennel, diced
4 oz. fresh sardine fillets
2 tablespoons white wine
1 teaspoon dried dill
Salt and pepper
2 oz. linguine pasta

Prep time: 5 min. / Cook time: 15 min. / Ready in: 20 min.

Heat the oil in a nonstick frying pan and sauté the onion. Add the garlic, diced fennel, sardine fillets, and white wine. Sprinkle with dill and salt and pepper. Remove garlic.
Meanwhile, cook the linguine in salted boiling water until al dente and drain. Top linguine with the sardine–fennel mixture and serve.

Bread

1 slice (1 oz.) whole grain bread

Cheese

½ cup (4 oz.) 1% milk fat cottage
cheese

Fruit

1 cup (6 oz.) fresh fruit salad

Gazpacho

1 cup (6 oz.) tomatoes, diced

¼ cup (2 oz.) red bell pepper,
diced

½ cup (2 oz.) cucumber, diced

¼ cup (2 oz.) onion, chopped

1 clove garlic, minced

2 basil leaves, chopped

2 tablespoons (1 oz.) wine vinegar

Dash Tabasco sauce

½ egg white

Salt and pepper, to taste

Prep time: 10 min. / Ready in: 10 min.

Mix ingredients in a blender on high for
4 minutes. Serve.

Spiced Lamb
with Carrots

4 oz. leg of lamb

1 teaspoon ground ginger

1 teaspoon ground nutmeg

1 cup (2 medium) diced carrots

Prep time: 10 min. / Cook time: 20 min. / Ready in: 30 min.

Season the leg of lamb with ginger
and nutmeg and grill or broil for about
20 minutes or as desired. Meanwhile, boil
or steam the carrots and mash them. Serve.

Yogurt

¾ cup (6 oz.) plain nonfat yogurt

Fruit

1 cup (6 oz.) fresh berries

GOURMET: PASTA

BREAKFAST

Hot Chocolate

Prep time: 2 min. / Cook time: 5 min. / Ready in: 7 min.

1 cup (8 fl. oz.) hot skim milk

2 tablespoons powdered hot
  chocolate mix

Put powdered chocolate mix in mug, add milk and stir. Microwave for 3–5 minutes or until hot. Stir and serve.

Ham Toast

Prep time: 2 min. / Cook time: 3 min. / Ready in: 5 min.

1 slice (1 oz.) whole grain bread

3 oz. smoked ham

Toast bread, top with ham, and serve.

LUNCH

Spaghetti with Pine Nuts

Prep time: 5 min. / Cook time: 15 min. / Ready in: 20 min.

2 oz. spaghetti

4 frozen artichoke hearts

¼ cup frozen peas

Salt and pepper

½ oz. (about 40) pine nuts

1 teaspoon olive oil

1 clove garlic, crushed

1 bunch basil, roughly chopped

2 tablespoons (1 oz.) grated
  Parmesan

1 bunch parsley, chopped

Cook spaghetti in salted boiling water until al dente. Drain and set aside. Blanch the artichoke hearts and peas in water for 5 minutes, then drain. Add a pinch of salt to season.

In a dry nonstick frying pan, toast the pine nuts until slightly golden brown; set aside. Add the olive oil and sauté garlic in the pan with the blanched artichoke hearts and peas for a minute. Add the cooked pasta, basil, pine nuts, and Parmesan cheese. Mix well and garnish with parsley. Serve.

Fruit

1 cup (6 oz.) fresh melon

Cumin Carrots

½ cup (4 fl. oz.) lemon juice

1 teaspoon ground cumin

1 cup (2 medium) grated carrots

Prep time: 5 min. / Ready in: 5 min.

Mix lemon juice and cumin and then pour over carrots. Serve.

Grilled Sea Bream Fillet with Eggplant

3 oz. sea bream fillet

1 medium eggplant, sliced

½ tablespoon lemon juice

Prep time: 20 min. / Cook time: 20 min. / Ready in: 40 min.

Heat oven to 350°F. Place eggplant in salted water for 20 minutes then drain, rinse, and dry. Bake the eggplant for 20 minutes or until tender. Meanwhile, grill, broil, or dry-fry the sea bream for 5–10 minutes or until flaky and season with lemon juice. Serve.

Yogurt

¾ cup (6 oz.) plain nonfat yogurt

Baked Pear

1 small pear, sliced in half and seeded

2 drops vanilla extract

Prep time: 2 min. / Cook time: 20 min. / Ready in: 22 min.

Preheat oven to 375°F. Place pear in baking dish, add a drop of vanilla extract to each half. Bake for 20 minutes or until tender. Serve.

BREAKFAST

Toast

1 slice (1 oz.) whole grain bread

Cook time: 2 min. / Ready in: 2 min.

Toast bread and serve.

Cheese

½ cup (4 oz.) 1% milk fat cottage cheese

Fruit

1 passionfruit

LUNCH

Mixed Salad

½ avocado
2 medium tomatoes
4 oz. shrimp
½ tablespoon balsamic vinegar

Prep time: 5 min. / Ready in: 5 min.

Chop the avocado and the tomatoes and mix with the shrimp. Season with balsamic vinegar. Serve.

Orechiette Pasta with Vegetables

1 (4 oz.) zucchini, peeled and cut into thin julienne strips
1 (3 oz.) carrot, peeled and cut into thin julienne strips
1 leek, peeled and cut into thin julienne strips
¼ cup (¾ oz.) snow peas
¼ cup (1 ½ oz.) diced yellow bell pepper
2 oz. orechiette pasta
3 teaspoons olive oil
2 tablespoons chopped parsley
Salt and pepper

Prep time: 10 min. / Cook time: 10 min. / Ready in: 20 min.

Blanch the vegetables in salted boiling water for 2 minutes then immediately plunge them into ice water to stop them from cooking further. Cook the pasta in salted boiling water for 8 minutes or until al dente. Heat the oil in a nonstick frying pan and sauté the chopped parsley. Add the vegetables. Drain pasta and add to vegetables. Add salt and pepper and mix thoroughly. Serve.

Yogurt

¾ cup (6 oz.) plain nonfat yogurt

Fruit

3 clementines

Vegetable Soup

1 cup (8 fl. oz.) fat-free vegetable soup (less than 100 calories per serving)

Cook time: 5 min. / Ready in: 5 min.

Heat soup in microwave or saucepan. Serve.

Chicken

4 oz. (4 slices) chicken breast deli meat

Cheese

¼ cup (2 oz.) part-skim ricotta cheese

Fruit

1 cup (6 oz.) lychees in light syrup, drained

GOURMET: PASTA

BREAKFAST

Yogurt

¾ cup (6 oz.) plain nonfat yogurt

Fruit

½ cup (4 oz.) applesauce with no
added sugar

LUNCH

Penne with Tomato, Pepper, and Feta Cheese

2 teaspoons olive oil

½ cup (3 oz.) red bell pepper,
diced

3 tablespoons Tomato Sauce (see
page 173)

2 oz. whole-wheat penne rigate

Salt and pepper

⅓ cup (2 oz.) crumbled reduced-
fat feta cheese

Prep time: 5 min. / Cook time: 15 min. / Ready in: 20 min.

In a frying pan, heat oil and fry the diced
pepper. Add the tomato sauce and cook for
5 minutes. Cook penne in salted boiling
water until al dente. Drain and add to sauce.
Season with salt and pepper and sprinkle
with feta cheese. Mix well and serve.

Fruit

1 cup (5 oz.) fresh watermelon
chunks

Shrimp and Spinach Salad

4 oz. cooked shrimp

1 large handful baby spinach leaves

1 tablespoon chopped mint

½ tablespoon lemon juice

Prep time: 5 min. / Ready in: 5 min.

Combine all ingredients and serve.

Peanut Butter Snack

1 teaspoon peanut butter

1 slice (1 oz.) whole grain bread

Prep time: 2 min. / Ready in: 2 min.

Spread peanut butter on bread (toasted if desired). Serve.

Cheese

1 slice (1 oz.) hard cheese (American, cheddar, Parmesan)

Fruit

1 small orange

BREAKFAST

Fruit

¾ cup (5 oz.) fruit in light syrup,
   drained

Milk

1 cup (8 fl. oz.) skim milk

LUNCH

Palm Salad

5 pieces (5 oz.) heart of palm
2 tablespoons Yogurt Dressing
   (see page 172)

Prep time: 2 min. / Ready in: 2 min.

Toss hearts of palm with dressing
and serve.

Ziti Pasta with Spinach and Cheese

3 cups (3 oz.) fresh spinach leaves
Salt and pepper
1 clove garlic, crushed
2 oz. ziti pasta
2 tablespoons (1 oz.) grated
   Parmesan cheese
1 teaspoon olive oil

Prep time: 5 min. / Cook time: 15 min. / Ready in: 20 min.

Wash the spinach, shake off most of the
water, and place in a nonstick frying pan.
Add salt and pepper and garlic. Cook for
10 minutes. Cook pasta in salted boiling
water until al dente. Remove spinach from
heat. Drain pasta and pour over spinach.
Stir in grated Parmesan and olive oil. Toss
together and serve.

Fruit

¾ cup (3 oz.) grapes

Egg Salad

2 medium eggs
1 teaspoon curry powder
1 large handful shredded lettuce
1 tablespoon chopped dill
1 serving Basic Vinaigrette
  (see page 170)

Prep time: 5 min. / Cook time: 5 min. / Ready in: 10 min.

Poach or dry-fry the eggs and sprinkle with curry powder. Toss the lettuce and dill and dress with the vinaigrette. Top with the eggs and serve.

Toast

1 slice (1 oz.) whole grain bread

Cook time: 2 min. / Ready in: 2 min.

Toast bread and serve.

Fruit

2 scoops (2 oz.) fruit sorbet

BREAKFAST

Soft-boiled Egg and Toast

1 medium egg
1 slice (1 oz.) whole grain bread

Prep time: 5 min. / Cook time: 6 min. / Ready in: 11 min.

Bring a saucepan half-filled with water to a boil. Reduce heat to a simmer, add egg, and cook for 3–6 minutes. Toast bread. Rinse egg under cold water and serve with toast.

Cheese

½ cup (4 oz.) 1% milk fat cottage cheese

LUNCH

Salad

¼ cup (2 oz.) cabbage, shredded
2 tablespoons Basic Vinaigrette (see page 170)

Prep time: 2 min. / Ready in: 2 min.

Toss cabbage with dressing and serve.

Spaghetti with Mussels and Zucchini

2 small (5 oz.) zucchini
4 oz. cooked shelled mussels
1 tablespoon olive oil
1 stalk celery, chopped
1 clove garlic, crushed
2 tablespoons white wine
Salt and pepper
1 tablespoon chopped parsley
2 oz. spaghetti

Prep time: 5 min. / Cook time: 15 min. / Ready in: 20 min.

Wash the zucchini and shave them into noodles with a peeler. Drain the mussels. In a large saucepan, heat the olive oil and sauté the celery and garlic. Add the mussels, zucchini noodles, wine, and salt and pepper; cook for 5 minutes, partly covered. Let cool slightly.
Cook the spaghetti in salted boiling water until al dente. Drain and pour over zucchini noodles and mussels. Add the chopped parsley. Mix and serve.

Fruit

1 kiwi

Gazpacho

1 cup (6 oz.) tomatoes, diced

¼ cup (2 oz.) red bell pepper, diced

½ cup (2 oz.) cucumber, diced

¼ cup (2 oz.) onion, chopped

1 clove garlic, minced

2 basil leaves, chopped

2 tablespoons (1 oz.) wine vinegar

Dash Tabasco sauce

½ egg white

Salt and pepper, to taste

Prep time: 10 min. / Ready in: 10 min.

Mix ingredients in a blender on high for 4 minutes. Serve.

Pork Chop and Mixed Vegetables

4 oz. lean boneless pork loin chop

1 teaspoon ground cinnamon

1 cup frozen mixed vegetables

Prep time: 5 min. / Cook time: 10 min. / Ready in: 15 min.

Grill or broil the pork chops for about 5 minutes or until no longer pink in center; sprinkle with cinnamon. Heat frozen vegetables in saucepan or microwave. Serve.

Fruit

1 cup (8 oz.) fresh strawberries

BREAKFAST

PB&J

Prep time: 2 min. / Cook time: 3 min. / Ready in: 5 min.

1 slice (1 oz.) whole grain bread
1 teaspoon peanut butter
2 teaspoons jam

Toast bread and spread with peanut butter and jam. Serve.

LUNCH

Mozzarella Salad

Prep time: 3 min. / Ready in: 3 min.

2 oz. light mozzarella
1 tablespoon balsamic vinegar

Slice the mozzarella, lightly sprinkle the vinegar over the top to taste.

Pasta Primavera

Prep time: 10 min. / Cook time: 10 min. / Ready in: 20 min.

½ cup (2 ½ oz.) zucchini
1 cup (6 oz.) cherry tomatoes
½ cup (1 ½ oz.) snow peas
½ cup (1 ½ oz.) sliced
  mushrooms
Salt and pepper
1 tablespoon olive oil
1 teaspoon lemon juice
2 oz. tagliatelle
Few sprigs parsley, chopped
1 bunch fresh chives, snipped

Wash zucchini, cherry tomatoes, snow peas, and mushrooms. Make zucchini noodles with a vegetable peeler. In a saucepan with half a glass of water, cook zucchini noodles, snow peas, mushrooms, and cherry tomatoes for 2 minutes. Add salt and pepper, olive oil, and lemon juice.
Cook the pasta in salted boiling water until al dente. Drain and place in a serving bowl. Add the vegetables and toss to combine. Sprinkle with pepper and the chopped herbs. Serve.

Fruit

1 cup (5 oz.) fresh fruit salad

Cucumber–Mint Gazpacho

1 cup (5 oz.) cucumber, diced
¼ cup (2 oz.) onion, chopped
1 clove garlic, minced
3 mint leaves, minced
2 tablespoons (1 oz.) wine vinegar
Dash Tabasco sauce
Salt and pepper, to taste

Prep time: 10 min. / Ready in: 10 min.

Mix ingredients in a blender on high for 4 minutes. Serve.

Grilled Catfish with Nutmeg and Soy Sauce

4 oz. catfish
Pinch of grated nutmeg
½ tablespoon soy sauce
½ cup (2 oz.) sliced carrots
½ cup (2 oz.) baby corn
1 tablespoon chopped cilantro

Prep time: 10 min. / Cook time: 15 min. / Ready in: 25 min.

Grill or dry-fry the catfish with the nutmeg and soy sauce until flaky. Steam the carrots and corn for 10 minutes and sprinkle with the cilantro. Serve.

Yogurt

¾ cup (6 oz.) plain nonfat yogurt

Fruit

1 stewed apple with cinnamon

BREAKFAST

Toast

1 slice (1 oz.) rye bread
2 teaspoons (⅓ oz.) butter

Cook time: 3 min. / Ready in: 3 min.

Toast bread and spread with butter. Serve.

Yogurt

¾ cup (6 oz.) plain nonfat yogurt

LUNCH

Avocado Salad

½ avocado
2 medium hard-boiled eggs
½ cup (2 oz.) fresh coleslaw
4 tablespoons Yogurt Dressing
(see page 172)

Prep time: 10 min. / Ready in: 10 min.

Combine ingredients and toss with dressing.

Yogurt

¾ cup (6 oz.) plain nonfat yogurt

Fruit

1 small pear

GOURMET: SANDWICH

Vegetable Soup

Cook time: 5 min. / Ready in: 5 min.

1 cup fat-free vegetable soup
(less than 100 calories per
serving)

Heat soup in microwave or saucepan. Serve.

Crab Sandwich

Prep time: 10 min. / Ready in: 10 min.

½ avocado
½ onion (red or white), chopped
Juice of ½ lemon
½ grapefruit
2 slices (2 oz.) rye bread
4 oz. flaked crab meat

Mash the avocado flesh and onion together, and add the lemon juice. Peel the grapefruit and cut into cubes. Spread the avocado mash on rye bread, and then add crab flakes and grapefruit cubes. Add another slice of rye bread. Serve.

Cheese

1 slice (1 oz.) cheddar cheese

BREAKFAST

Toast

Prep time: 1 min. / Cook time: 3 min. / Ready in: 4 min

1 slice (1 oz.) walnut bread
2 teaspoons jam

Toast bread and spread with jam. Serve.

Cheese

½ cup (4 oz.) 1% milk fat cottage
  cheese

LUNCH

Bacon Salad

Prep time: 2 min. / Cook time: 8 min. / Ready in: 10 min.

4 slices Canadian bacon
Handful shredded lettuce
1 tablespoon balsamic vinegar

Dry-fry the bacon, let cool. Crumble bacon over lettuce, and toss with balsamic vinegar. Serve.

Goat Cheese Sandwich

Prep time: 10 min. / Ready in: 10 min.

4 oz. fresh goat cheese
2 tablespoons (1 oz.) light sour
  cream
2 slices (2 oz.) whole grain bread
1 sprig fresh thyme, leaves
  chopped

Mix cheese and sour cream. Spread over the bread and grill for a few minutes in the toaster oven. Sprinkle with thyme and serve.

Fruit

2 tangerines

GOURMET: SANDWICH

Chicken Breast and Vegetables

4 oz. chicken breast

½ tablespoon soy sauce

⅝ cup (2 ½ oz.) bean sprouts

½ cup (2 oz.) sliced bamboo shoots

¼ cup (2 oz.) broccoli florets

Yogurt

¾ cup (6 oz.) plain nonfat yogurt

Fruit

1 kiwi

Prep time: 10 min. / Cook time: 15 min. / Ready in: 25 min.

Season chicken with soy sauce and grill or dry-fry until opaque at center. Steam the vegetables for 10 minutes. Serve.

GOURMET: SANDWICH

Breakfast

Pastry

1 small (2 ½ oz.) sweet roll (less
than 150 kcal per serving)

Milk

1 cup (8 fl. oz.) skim milk

Lunch

Tomato–Mozzarella
Salad

½ cup (3 oz.) tomatoes, sliced
2 oz. mozzarella
½ tablespoon balsamic vinegar

Prep time: 5 min. / Ready in: 5 min.

Combine ingredients. Serve.

Yogurt

¾ cup (6 oz.) nonfat yogurt

Fruit

1 slice (5 oz.) mango

Leeks

2 leeks, sliced lengthwise

Prep time: 5 min. / Cook time: 10 min. / Ready in: 15 min.

Steam leeks for about 8 minutes or until tender. Serve.

Open Vegetarian Sandwich

2 slices (2 oz.) pumpernickel bread

1 teaspoon olive oil

1 teaspoon Dijon mustard

1 tablespoon lemon juice

1 large handful salad leaves, chopped

5 radishes (3 oz.) , finely sliced

1 small (1 oz.) tomato, finely sliced

¼ cup (1 oz.) cucumber, peeled, seeded, and finely sliced

2 medium hard-boiled eggs, sliced

1 tablespoon capers

Salt and pepper

Prep time: 10 min. / Ready in: 10 min.

Toast bread. Combine oil, mustard, and lemon juice. Finely slice salad leaves, radishes, tomato, and cucumber. Layer the vegetables on top of the toast slices, starting with the lettuce. Drizzle with dressing. Complete with egg slices, capers, and salt and pepper. Serve.

Yogurt

¾ cup (6 oz.) plain nonfat yogurt

Fruit

1 small orange

BREAKFAST

Cereal

Prep time: 2 min. / Ready in: 2 min.

2–3 tablespoons (1 oz.) unfrosted
whole grain cereal

1 cup (8 fl. oz.) skim milk

Pour cereal and milk into bowl, serve.

Nuts

6 almonds

Milk

1 cup (8 fl. oz.) skim milk

LUNCH

Salad

Prep time: 2 min. / Ready in: 2 min.

Handful shredded lettuce

4 tablespoons Basic Vinaigrette
(see page 170)

Toss lettuce with vinaigrette dressing and
serve.

Omelet

2 medium eggs

Prep time: 2 min. / Cook time: 8 min. / Ready in: 10 min.

Yogurt

Whisk eggs, heat in a dry nonstick frying
pan over medium heat, stirring frequently.
Serve.

¾ cup (6 oz.) plain nonfat
yogurt

Fruit

½ grapefruit

Tomato Soup

Cook time: 5 min. / Ready in: 5 min.

1 cup (8 fl. oz.) tomato soup (less than 100 calories per serving)

Heat in saucepan or microwave. Serve.

Parmesan Panini

Prep time: 1 hour 15 min. / Ready in: 1 hour 15 min.

4 oz. lean beef carpaccio

1 teaspoon chopped basil

Juice of ¼ lemon

Salt and pepper

1 teaspoon capers

2 oz. whole wheat hot dog bun

2 lettuce leaves

2 tablespoons (1 oz.) Parmesan shavings

Place meat in freezer for 1 hour, then place on dish. Combine basil and lemon juice and pour over meat. Season with salt and pepper, sprinkle with capers, and marinate for at least 10 minutes. Toast the hot dog bun and layer it with lettuce, carpaccio, and Parmesan shavings. Serve.

or

Swedish Sandwich

Prep time: 10 min. / Ready in: 10 min.

½ cup (4 oz.) 1% milk fat cottage cheese

¼ cup (1 oz./half a small) cucumber, diced

1 teaspoon lemon juice

2 oz. whole wheat bun

4 oz. smoked salmon

Few sprigs of dill

Mix cottage cheese with diced cucumber and lemon juice. Split and toast the bun, then spread with the cucumber cream. Cut the salmon into thin slices and arrange on the bread. Garnish with dill sprigs. Serve.

Sorbet

2 scoops (2 oz.) fruit sorbet

GOURMET: SANDWICH

BREAKFAST

Toast

1 slice (1 oz.) whole grain bread

Cook time: 3 min. / Ready in: 3 min.

Toast bread and serve.

Fresh Fruit Smoothie

Juice of 1 clementine

1 clementine, peeled and seeded

1 small apple, peeled, seeded, and chopped

1 cup (2 oz.) carrot, peeled and grated

Juice of 1 lemon

1 cup (8 fl. oz.) skim milk

1 teaspoon sweetener

Prep time: 3 min. / Ready in: 3 min.

Combine all the ingredients in a blender and blend until smooth and creamy. Serve chilled or with ice.

Cheese

1 slice (1 oz.) hard cheese (American, cheddar, Parmesan)

LUNCH

Chicken Salad

4 oz. diced chicken breast

1 cup (2 oz.) carrot, grated

1 cup (2 oz.) celery, diced

2 tablespoons Yogurt Dressing (see page 172)

Prep time: 3 min. / Cook time: 10 min. / Ready in: 13 min.

Grill or broil the chicken breast for 10 minutes or until opaque in center. Toss chicken, carrots, and celery with dressing. Serve.

Fruit

1 small pear

Zucchini Soup

Cook time: 5 min. / Ready in: 5 min.

1 cup (8 fl. oz.) zucchini soup (less than 100 calories per serving)

Heat in saucepan or microwave. Serve.

Tuna and Egg Sandwich

Prep time: 10 min. / Ready in: 10 min.

1 onion, chopped

2 oz. tuna packed in water, drained

1 teaspoon Dijon mustard

½ cup (4 oz.) 1% milk fat cottage cheese

½ tablespoon lemon juice

Salt and pepper

2 slices (2 oz.) Italian bread

1 medium hard-boiled egg

1 sprig parsley, chopped

Mix the onion, tuna, mustard, cottage cheese, and lemon juice. Add salt and pepper. Spread the mixture over the bread. Add the sliced hard-boiled egg and parsley. Serve.

or

Swedish Sandwich
(see page 237)

Fruit

1 kiwi

GOURMET: SANDWICH

Breakfast

Bagel

½ whole grain bagel

Cook time: 5 min. / Ready in: 5 min.

Toast bagel and serve.

Yogurt

2 teaspoons honey
¾ cup (6 oz.) plain nonfat yogurt

Prep time: 1 min. / Ready in: 1 min.

Mix honey in yogurt and serve.

Lunch

Oven-baked Tilapia with Mixed Vegetables

2 scallions, chopped
1 tablespoon sliced ginger root
½ teaspoon red chili flakes
4 oz. tilapia (or other fish)
2 tablespoons white wine
1 cup (3 oz.) frozen mixed
  vegetables

Prep time: 10 min. / Cook time: 30 min. / Ready in: 40 min.

Preheat oven to 400°F. Mix the scallions, ginger, and chili flakes and place them on a square of parchment paper in a baking dish. Rinse the fish well inside and out, pat dry, season lightly with salt, and place on top of the mixture. Add the wine and close the parchment paper into a parcel. Bake for 15 minutes, then rotate the pan once and continue cooking for an additional 10–15 minutes, until a fork easily enters the thickest part of the fish.

Meanwhile, heat the vegetables in a saucepan or microwave. Transfer the fish to a warm dish with the sauce and serve with mixed vegetables.

Yogurt

¾ cup (6 oz.) plain nonfat yogurt

Fruit

1 diced apple with cinnamon

GOURMET: SANDWICH

Pumpkin Soup

1 cup (8 fl. oz.) pumpkin soup
(less than 100 calories per
serving)

Cook time: 5 min. / Ready in: 5 min.

Heat in a saucepan or microwave. Serve.

Rustic Sandwich

2 onions, sliced

4 oz. thinly sliced liver

2 slices (2 oz.) whole-wheat
bread

Salt and pepper

Prep time: 5 min. / Cook time: 5 min. / Ready in: 10 min.

Cook the onions in the microwave with a few drops of water for 3 minutes or until soft. Fry the slices of liver in a nonstick frying pan for 5 minutes and add the onions. Top the bread with the liver and onions. Season with salt and pepper to taste. Serve.

Cheese

¼ cup (2 oz.) part-skim ricotta
cheese

Fruit

1 cup (6 oz.) fresh fruit salad

Breakfast

Toast

1 slice (1 oz.) whole grain bread

2 teaspoons jam

Cook time: 3 min. / Ready in: 3 min.

Toast bread, spread with jam, and serve.

Yogurt

¾ cup (6 oz.) plain nonfat yogurt

Lunch

Hamburger with Vegetables

4 oz. lean ground beef

1 cup mixed vegetables

1 teaspoon ketchup

Prep time: 2 min. / Cook time: 10 min. / Ready in: 12 min.

Grill or dry-fry the hamburger for 10 minutes or as desired. Steam the vegetables. Serve hamburger with ketchup and steamed vegetables.

Cheese

¼ cup (2 oz.) part-skim
  ricotta cheese

Fruit

1 cup (5 oz.) fresh pineapple
  chunks

GOURMET: SANDWICH

Noodle Soup

1 cup Ramen noodles (less than
    100 calories per serving)

Cook time: 5 min. / Ready in: 5 min.

Heat in a saucepan or microwave per package instructions. Serve.

Curried Chicken Sandwich

4 oz. chicken breast

⅓ cup (3 oz.) plain nonfat yogurt

1 teaspoon curry powder

Lettuce leaves, shredded

2 slices (2 oz.) whole-wheat
    bread with raisins

Prep time: 5 min. / Cook time: 10 min. / Ready in: 15 min.

Dry-fry chicken in a nonstick frying pan for 5 minutes or until opaque in center. Remove and shred finely. Mix the yogurt with the curry powder then add the chicken. Place the lettuce on the bread and top with chicken. Sprinkle with a little more curry powder. Serve.

Yogurt

⅓ cup (3 oz.) plain nonfat yogurt

Fruit

8 fresh lychees

GOURMET: SANDWICH

BREAKFAST

Toast

1 slice (1 oz.) whole grain bread
2 teaspoons (⅓ oz.) butter

Cook time: 3 min. / Ready in: 3 min.

Toast bread, spread with butter, and serve.

Yogurt

¾ cup (6 oz.) plain nonfat yogurt

Fruit

1 cup fresh orange juice

LUNCH

Mediterranean Salad

½ avocado
1 medium hard-boiled egg
1 cup (6 oz.) diced tomatoes
½ cup (2 oz./1 small) cucumber, diced
2 tablespoons Basic Vinaigrette (see page 170)

Prep time: 10 min. / Ready in: 10 min.

Combine ingredients. Serve.

Yogurt

¾ cup (6 oz.) plain nonfat yogurt

Fruit

1 small pear

Tomato Chickpeas

Prep time: 3 min. / Ready in: 3 min.

½ cup chickpeas, canned or cooked

3 tablespoons Tomato Sauce (see page 173)

Mix together and serve.

Stuffed Peppers

Prep time: 10 min. / Cook time: 60 min. / Ready in: 70 min.

2 green bell peppers

⅓ cup (2 oz.) brown rice

4 tomatoes, diced

2 onions, chopped

1 medium egg

Salt and pepper

2 tablespoons (1 oz.) light sour cream

1 tablespoon chopped parsley

Preheat oven to 400°F. Slice off the top of the peppers like a cap, remove seeds, and blanch for 3 minutes.

Rinse rice and put in a saucepan with 1 cup water; bring to a boil over high heat. Reduce heat to low and cover, allowing rice to simmer for 20 minutes. Turn heat off and let rice sit for an additional 10 minutes. Meanwhile, heat diced tomatoes and chopped onions in a dry, nonstick frying pan until softened, or heat in the microwave for 3 minutes. Beat the egg and mix with the tomatoes and onions into the rice. Season with salt and pepper. Stuff the peppers with the mixture, top with sour cream. Bake for 30 minutes. Garnish with parsley and serve.

Prep time: 5 min. / Ready in: 5 min.

Strawberry Smoothie

1 cup (8 fl. oz.) skim milk

1 cup (8 oz.) fresh strawberries

Blend milk and strawberries together until smooth and serve.

GOURMET: VEGETARIAN

BREAKFAST

PB&J Toast

Cook time: 3 min. / Ready in: 3 min.

1 slice (1 oz.) whole grain bread
3 teaspoons peanut butter
2 teaspoons jam

Toast bread, spread with peanut butter and jam. Serve.

Cheese

½ cup (4 oz.) 1% milk fat cottage cheese

LUNCH

Vegetable Patties with Steamed Vegetables

Prep time: 5 min. / Cook time: 15 min. / Ready in: 20 min.

2 vegetarian patties
2–3 cups mixed vegetables (tomatoes, carrots, broccoli, etc.)

Dry-fry the patties for 15 minutes (or per package instructions) while steaming the vegetables or heating them in the microwave. Serve.

Yogurt

¾ cup (6 oz.) plain nonfat yogurt

Fruit

1 apple

GOURMET: VEGETARIAN

Black Beans and Mushroom Tortillas

1 onion, minced

1 cup (2 ½ oz.) mushrooms, diced

1 tomato, chopped

1 teaspoon olive oil

½ cup cooked black beans

2 stalks celery, chopped

1 tablespoon soy sauce

½ teaspoon chopped sage

Salt and pepper

2 whole-wheat soft tortillas (6-inch diameter)

Prep time: 5 min. / Cook time: 23 min. / Ready in: 28 min.

Preheat oven to 375°F. Fry the onion, mushrooms, and tomato in olive oil. Add to a baking dish with the black beans, celery, and soy sauce. Bake for 10 minutes, then season with sage and salt and pepper. Stuff and roll the tortillas with the mixture and return to the oven for 10 minutes to warm. Serve.

Yogurt

¾ cup (6 oz.) plain nonfat yogurt

Fruit

1 kiwi

GOURMET: VEGETARIAN

BREAKFAST

Whole Grain Toast

1 slice (1 oz.) whole grain bread

2 teaspoons (⅓ oz.) butter

Cook time: 3 min. / Ready in: 3 min.

Toast bread, spread with butter, and serve.

Hot Chocolate

1 cup (8 fl. oz.) hot skim milk

2 tablespoons powdered hot chocolate mix

Prep time: 2 min. / Cook time: 5 min. / Ready in: 7 min.

Put powdered chocolate mix in mug, add milk and stir. Microwave for 3–5 minutes or until hot. Stir and serve.

LUNCH

Mozzarella, Tomato, and Corn Salad

2 medium tomatoes, chopped

2 oz. light mozzarella cheese, sliced

½ cup canned corn kernels

2 tablespoons Basic Vinaigrette (see page 170)

Prep time: 10 min. / Ready in: 10 min.

Combine all the ingredients and serve.

Yogurt

¾ cup (6 oz.) plain nonfat yogurt

Fruit

1 slice (5 oz.) mango

Leeks

2 leeks, sliced lengthwise

2 tablespoons Basic Vinaigrette
(see page 170)

Prep time: 5 min. / Cook time: 8 min. / Ready in: 13 min.

Steam the leeks for 8 minutes or until tender. Dress with vinaigrette and serve.

Asparagus Flan

2 slices (2 oz.) white bread

¼ cup (2 fl. oz.) skim milk

5 oz. (about 10 medium) green
asparagus spears, trimmed

1 medium egg, beaten

Salt and pepper

Pinch of nutmeg

Few sprigs of chervil, chopped

Prep time: 5 min. / Cook time: 40 min. / Ready in: 45 min.

Preheat oven to 375°F. Soak bread in a little of the milk. Steam asparagus for 10 minutes or until tender and drain. Set aside 5 asparagus spears. Cut the remaining spears into small pieces and mash with the bread. Add egg and remaining milk. Add salt and pepper, nutmeg, and chervil. Pour the batter into a nonstick baking pan and garnish with the reserved asparagus spears. Bake for 30 minutes. Serve.

Cheese

1 slice (1 oz.) hard cheese
(American, cheddar, Parmesan)

Fruit

1 orange

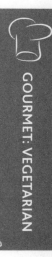

BREAKFAST

Pancake

Prep time: 2 min. / Ready in: 2 min.

1 pancake

1 tablespoon maple syrup

Heat pancake, top with maple syrup, serve.

Yogurt

¾ cup (6 oz.) plain nonfat yogurt

LUNCH

Salad

Prep time: 5 min. / Ready in: 5 min.

2 cups salad greens and
  vegetables of your choice,
  chopped

2 tablespoons Yogurt Dressing
  (see page 172)

Toss salad vegetables with dressing and
serve.

Grilled Cheese Sandwich

Prep time: 2 min. / Cook time: 3 min. / Ready in: 5 min.

2 slices (2 oz.) hard cheese
  (American, cheddar, Parmesan)

2 slices (2 oz.) whole grain bread

Place the cheese slices on the bread and
grill in toaster oven until melted. Serve.

Milk

1 cup (8 fl. oz.) skim milk

Fruit

1 orange

Lentil and Vegetable Salad

¼ cup dry lentils (for ½ cup cooked)

¼ cup (2 oz.) diced tomatoes

¼ cup (½ medium) grated carrot

¼ cup (½ oz.) baby corn

1 tablespoon chopped cilantro

1 serving Tomato Citrus Vinaigrette (see page 171)

Prep time: 15 min. / Cook time: 20 min. / Ready in: 35 min.

Rinse lentils. Bring to a boil with ¾ cup water in a saucepan over high heat, reduce heat and simmer for about 20 minutes or until lentils are tender. Combine all the ingredients, toss with vinaigrette, and serve.

Yogurt

¾ cup (6 oz.) plain nonfat yogurt

Applesauce

1 apple, peeled, cored, and diced

Cinnamon

Prep time: 3 min. / Cook time: 15 min. / Ready in: 18 min.

Cook apple with ½ cup water in a saucepan over high heat for about 15 minutes or until tender. Mash and sprinkle with cinnamon to taste. Serve.

BREAKFAST

Toast

Cook time: 3 min. / Ready in: 3 min.

1 slice (1 oz.) French bread

2 teaspoons (⅓ oz.) butter

Toast bread, spread with butter, and serve.

Yogurt

¾ cup (6 oz.) plain nonfat yogurt

Fruit

1 apple

LUNCH

Mushroom Omelet

Prep time: 5 min. / Cook time: 10 min. / Ready in: 13 min.

½ cup (1 oz.) sliced mushrooms

2 medium eggs

2 tablespoons (1 oz.) light sour cream

2 tablespoons (1 oz.) grated Parmesan cheese

Heat the mushrooms in nonstick frying pan over medium heat. Meanwhile, whisk the eggs, sour cream, and Parmesan cheese together. Add to mushrooms and cook a for about 8 minutes.

Fruit

1 small banana

Beet and Chickpea Salad

1 medium cooked beet, diced

½ cup canned chickpeas, drained

2 tablespoons Basic Vinaigrette (see page 170)

Prep time: 10 min. / Ready in: 10 min.

Toss vegetables with vinaigrette and serve.

Pita Pizza

1 (2 oz.) whole-wheat pita bread

3 tablespoons Tomato Sauce (see page 173)

2 medium tomatoes, sliced

1 onion, sliced

3 tablespoons black olives, halved

2 tablespoons (1 oz.) grated Parmesan cheese

1 tablespoon dried oregano, crushed

Prep time: 5 min. / Cook time: 15 min. / Ready in: 20 min.

Preheat oven to 400°F. Split pita bread in half. Spread a little tomato sauce on each half. Add tomatoes, onions, olives, cheese, and oregano. Bake for 15 minutes. Serve.

Fruit

½ grapefruit

GOURMET: VEGETARIAN

Breakfast

Cereal

2–3 tablespoons (1 oz.) unfrosted
  whole grain cereal
1 cup (8 fl. oz.) skim milk

Prep time: 2 min. / Ready in: 2 min.

Pour cereal and milk into bowl, serve.

Milk

1 cup (8 fl. oz.) skim milk

Nuts

6 nuts

Fruit

1 kiwi

Lunch

Mixed Garden Salad

1 large handful lettuce
½ cup (3 ¾ oz./1 small)
  cucumber, diced
1 handful cherry tomatoes,
  halved
2 oz. vegan jerky
¼ cup (1 oz.) diced hard cheese
2 tablespoons Yogurt Dressing
  (see page 172)

Prep time: 15 min. / Ready in: 15 min.

Combine all the ingredients and serve.

Fruit

1 cup (5 oz.) fresh pineapple
  chunks

Vegetarian Chili

1 onion, diced

¼ tablespoon ground cumin

¼ teaspoon ground cayenne
pepper

1 teaspoon olive oil

2 cloves garlic, crushed

1 cup (2 medium) green bell
peppers, seeded and diced

1 can peeled tomatoes

½ cup canned red kidney beans,
drained

⅓ cup (2 oz.) canned corn
kernels, drained

Salt and pepper

Few leaves cilantro, minced

Prep time: 5 min. / Cook time: 20 min. / Ready in: 25 min.

In a nonstick frying pan, sauté chopped onions and spices in olive oil for 1 minute. Add garlic and bell peppers, and cook for 1 minute. Stir in tomatoes and 1 cup water and bring to a boil. Add beans and corn. Simmer for 15 minutes. Season with salt and pepper. Garnish with cilantro and serve.

Cheese

1 oz. hard cheese (American,
cheddar, Parmesan)

Sorbet

2 scoops (2 oz.) strawberry sorbet

BREAKFAST

Gouda Crispbreads

Prep time: 2 min. / Ready in: 2 min.

2 reduced-fat crispbread crackers
(about 1 oz.)

1 slice (1 oz.) Gouda cheese

Top crispbreads with Gouda, serve.

Nuts

12 almonds

Fruit

1 cup (4 oz.) grapes

LUNCH

Noodles

Prep time: 5 min. / Cook time: 4 min. / Ready in: 9 min.

½ cup (4 oz.) dry Ramen noodles
(for 1 ½ cup cooked)

½ cup canned kidney beans,
drained

1 cup (3 oz.) frozen Chinese
stir-fry vegetables

1 teaspoon sesame oil

Add noodles to 1 cup salted boiling water, cook about 4 minutes (or per package instructions). Meanwhile, heat vegetables in a saucepan or microwave. Combine all the ingredients and serve.

Yogurt

¾ cup (6 oz.) plain nonfat yogurt

Fruit

8 fresh lychees

Carrot Salad

2 medium carrots

Lemon juice, to taste

Prep time: 3 min. / Ready in: 3 min.

Peel and grate carrots, season with lemon juice, and serve.

Fried Tofu with Green Peppers

4 oz. firm tofu, drained and cubed

1 teaspoon sesame oil

2 medium green bell peppers, chopped

3 tablespoons soy sauce

Salt and pepper

Prep time: 5 min. / Cook time: 8 min. / Ready in: 13 min.

Fry tofu in oil in a nonstick frying pan until cooked through. Add green peppers, soy sauce, and salt and pepper. Stir, cover, and simmer for 5–6 minutes. Serve.

Yogurt

½ cup (4 oz.) nonfat fruit yogurt

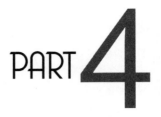

PART 4

YOUR RIGHT WEIGHT
FOR LIFE

CHAPTER 9

DINING OUT

W HEN YOU ARE ON A DIET, it's hard to imagine putting yourself in temptation's way by accepting an invitation to eat out; it may feel like you're setting yourself up for a night of torture. And it's just as easy to feel guilty for pulling into a fast food restaurant or gorging on pizza. We all have moments of weakness. But if you plan for these situations in advance, you can have solutions ready to help make good choices when eating on the run. For example, it's wise to have a glass of water alongside your wine and keep it on the right-hand side of your wine glass; it's a safe bet that your hand will drift to the water, saving you 70 calories. No matter what, don't abandon your social life just because you're dieting; follow these pointers for ordering at different kinds of restaurants. And remember that the biggest obstacle you'll face when eating out is portion size—stop eating when you're full and take home the leftovers!

AMERICAN

As an appetizer, choose either one thin slice of smoked salmon with a piece of unbuttered toast; or six oysters or as much other shellfish (except oysters) as you want with two teaspoons of cocktail sauce or vinaigrette; or a small salad of your choice. For the main course, order four ounces meat or equivalent, preferably grilled or steamed with two tablespoons sauce; *and* mixed greens; *and* four tablespoons limited starch (see page 77) or two slices of bread. For dessert choose between a five-ounce glass of wine; *or* two golf ball-sized scoops of sorbet; *or* one half of a piece of pie.

CHINESE

For your appetizer, choose either four steamed shrimp, beef, or crab dumplings; *or* soup plus three steamed dumplings; *or* a spring roll along with a crab or shrimp salad. Order as your main course four ounces meat or any other equivalent with two tablespoons sauce; *and* sautéed vegetables; *and* a small bowl of plain rice. Choose either two golfball sized scoops (2 oz.) of sorbet; *or* twelve fresh lychees; *or* one slice of mango or pineapple for dessert.

FRENCH

For an appetizer, choose the French onion soup *or* salmon tartare *or* toasted goat cheese salad *or niçoise salad* (tuna, eggs, and black olives). For the main course, order a hanger steak with black peppercorn sauce *or coq au vin* or Beef Bourguignon (beef stew) *or* mussels in a white wine and garlic sauce. You can choose between either one or two (5 oz.) glasses of wine *or* a dessert. If you choose dessert, select two scoops (2 oz.) of homemade sorbet, *or* chocolate mousse, *or* a poached pear with chocalate sauce, *or* a slice of fruit pie.

ITALIAN

Avoid sauces such as Alfredo and carbonara, which are made with heavy cream and are rich in fat. Also, steer clear of the Parmigiana dishes (eggplant, chicken, veal, etc.), as these are breaded, fried, and topped with cheese. Instead go with a light red sauce on pasta and have a salad as an accompaniment. Restrict yourself to a moderate amount of cheese on your Italian dishes, and choose grilled meat, fish, or poultry for your main course.

Japanese

When we think of Japanese cuisine, we think of sushi. Yes, it can be healthy, but remember that the rice is usually flavored with salt, vinegar, and sugar, adding hidden calories. Plus, sushi is served in bite-size portions, so it is easy to overeat without realizing you are doing so. Slow down and savor each bite. For an appetizer, order a miso soup. For the main course, choose between ten sashimi; *or* ten sushi; *or* ten maki. As dessert, choose either fruit salad; *or* two golfball sized scoops (2 oz.) of matcha green tea sorbet.

Mexican

Rice, beans, and tortillas can be healthy and filling, as long as they're not loaded with cheese and sour cream. A tostada with a low-fat cheese is a good option. Choose a spicy salsa to add flavor, without a lot of calories, to your meal.

Fast Food

If you're in a hurry, just order carefully. Here's how:

- **Burgers/Chicken**

A regular cheeseburger with condiments (300 calories), plus a side salad with one tablespoon low-fat balsamic vinaigrette (55 calories), a fruit yogurt (160 calories), and a bottle of water or a can of diet soda (zero calories); or six chicken nuggets (280 calories), plus a side salad with one tablespoon low-fat balsamic vinaigrette (55 calories), two apple slices (30 calories), 1% low-fat milk (100 calories). The worst culprits at fast-food chains are the side orders such as French fries and sweetened sodas, not the burgers.

- **Pizza**

If you're dying for a slice of pizza, you can replace a diet plan lunch with one slice, followed by a piece of fruit. Be aware, however, that pizza has a low satiety level. Choose an independent pizzeria as opposed to one that is part of a large chain, and order a traditional thin-crust pizza. Opt for a Margherita (tomato, basil, and mozzarella) or vegetarian pizza without many toppings. Ask the restaurant to go easy on the cheese, and avoid eating the crust, which equals an extra portion of bread

• **Sandwiches**

If your only option is to make or order a quick sandwich, that's fine. Don't beat yourself up. Take two slices of whole grain or rye bread; or one pita bread. Add four ounces lean meat (ham, beef, chicken) or tuna in brine, or two medium hard-boiled eggs, or two ounces hard cheese (cheddar or Swiss) or mozzarella. Add as many vegetables you like (tomatoes and lettuce) as well as lemon juice, mustard, and pickles. Skip butter, margarine, mayonnaise, and olive oil. Eat your sandwich with a piece of fruit. This will provide extra sugar, increase your intake of fiber, and help keep you feeling satisfied until dinner.

CHAPTER 10

CRAVINGS AND OTHER STUMBLING BLOCKS

We all struggle when dieting. Below are some common roadblocks, along with tips on how to beat them and move on.

I'M HUNGRY

True hunger is a sign of good health. It's normal to feel hungry before a meal. And in the early days of a weight-loss diet you will obviously feel more hungry than usual. Happily, this does not last long and the feeling gradually subsides. It is also normal to feel slightly hungry even after having eaten because satiety signals take five to ten minutes to reach the brain.

However, as hunger pangs do exist and are not pleasant, you need to learn to counter them aggressively. Drink water, unsweetened tea or coffee, and diet sodas. If this is insufficient, turn to nourishing food. Always start with less rich foods: a nonfat yogurt or a piece of fruit or two. If you're continuously plagued by hunger pangs, prepare raw vegetables in advance—cauliflower, carrot sticks, or cherry tomatoes—along with a dip made of nonfat plain yogurt, flavored with salt, pepper, and herbs. You can eat as much of this as you wish. It's important to have these snacks ready. If they're already prepared, you're less likely to head for a chunk of cheese or candy bar.

If you are still hungry after these healthy snacks, then go ahead and eat a small amount of whatever it is you are craving. Make smart food choices: for example, chomping on an apple will be a lot more satisfying than sipping an apple juice. You should never stay frustrated, but moderation is essential when you feed a craving or stray from the menus. Little by little, you will learn to refocus your hunger. You will soon realize that a yogurt or a piece of fruit is enough, and pretty soon you will no longer even need those.

I Want Wine, Chocolate, and Bread

The three most common cravings are for a glass of wine, chocolate, and bread. Waging war against all three is completely futile.

If you really want to drink wine with a meal, limit yourself to one five-ounce glass. Have the wine in place of the fruit for that meal.

You can do the same sort of swap with chocolate. Three normal-size squares of chocolate weigh about a half an ounce and have approximately the same number of calories as a piece of fruit. However, if you can be satisfied with a single square of chocolate per day, there's no need to deprive yourself: 30 additional calories a day is not going to threaten the balance of your diet.

Although you can eat bread in the Gourmet phase of this diet, it is more difficult to find an equivalent for it in the other phases. If you really can't do without bread, replace an ounce of cheese or a nonfat plain yogurt with a slice (1 oz.) of bread.

I Love Pasta!

In the Gourmet phase of this diet, you can have three and a half ounces of carbohydrates every evening. If that portion size seems too small then eat your carbohydrate ration every other day so you can double it. And remember, stick to plain red tomato sauce. As soon as you add oil, butter, cream, or cheese, you risk going off the rails. Cooked al dente or in its whole-wheat version, pasta gives lasting energy. By avoiding drops in blood sugar levels, you avoid sugar cravings!

My Kitchen is a Diet Trap

Unless you take time to evaluate what's in your cupboards before you begin your diet, you're asking for trouble. Of course you should get rid of unhealthy temptation, but you should also stock up on healthy basics. Your refrigerator should contain nonfat dairy products, your pantry should have canned vegetables, and make sure there's some meat in the freezer. Always keep eggs in your fridge. If possible, buy cheese in individual one ounce portions. Buy small containers of pureed fruit or cook fruit without sugar, with or without the addition of spices.

If your family is not on the diet with you, temptations abound. Reserve a shelf in the pantry and, if possible, in the fridge exclusively for the foods that you're allowed. That way you will acquire the reflex of looking only in "your area" when you have an urge to eat.

I'm a Snackaholic!

Snacking is more of a habit than a need and therefore you simply need to get out of the habit. Sometimes you only need to change the way you prepare food to make it more appealing. Instead of just crunching on an apple, cut it up into small cubes and sprinkle on a little ground cinnamon.

This Tastes Bland

Seasoning your meat and fish will transform the flavor of the dish. A few well-chosen herbs sprinkled over meat before you broil it will give it a whole new taste. Cook fish in a parchment or foil parcel with some tomatoes, a little onion, fresh ground pepper, and curry powder to give your palate a treat.

I'm Tired

It is not uncommon to feel tired when dieting; taking a multivitamin to make up for any potential deficiencies should help.

THE RECOVERY PLAN

There will inevitably be times when you find you just can't stick to your diet plan. Allow yourself these breaks, but just be sure you have a recovery plan to make up for your indulgence. If you have a large meal one evening or an extra cocktail or a rich dessert, simply replace one of the two meals the next day with the following:

- 2 medium hard-boiled eggs (whites only, no yolk)

- unlimited quantities of raw vegetables or steamed green vegetables, cooked without fat

- 1 nonfat yogurt (without sugar; with sweetener if desired) or 1 cup (8 fl. oz.) nonfat milk

Don't add any fruit, starches, or fat with this recovery plan meal.

If you have a special occasion coming up or you know you're likely to go over your diet plan limits at a subsequent meal, you can even use the recovery plan in advance. You can use this recovery plan meal as necessary, but I recommend that you restrict it to a maximum of twice a week in order to maintain the necessary nutritional balance over the course of the week.

Note: this recovery plan is **not** advisable for **diabetics**. Instead, after a break from a diet phase, diabetics should return to their previous diet phase and increase physical activity by an additional fifteen minutes per day (walking, swimming, biking, etc.) for a duration of two weeks.

Chapter 11

BON APPÉTIT!

You Did It!

Congratulations, you have reached your Right Weight target and now it's time to return to a normal diet. The most important thing to keep in mind is the difference between unrestricted meals and eating excessively. An unrestricted meal is one where you choose two of its components (appetizer, main course, or dessert) and eat what you'd like for those two components. But you keep the third component light: for instance, a salad with just a tablespoon of oil for the appetizer or a piece of fruit for the dessert. A meal becomes excessive if you have more than two unrestricted courses.

Unrestricted Meals

Put the following strategy into place for gradually increasing the number of unrestricted meals you consume. For the first two weeks, continue your diet as you've been doing, but have three unrestricted meals each week. For the following two weeks, increase this number to five per week. Your weight should stabilize. Continue to increase the number of unrestricted meals until you are eating nine unrestricted meals and five low-calorie meals from the diet plan per week. Once you have reached this stage, stay there. **Continue eating five low-calorie meals per week. There is no other way to maintain your weight loss.**

Stay On Track

Those who have been overweight in the past may gradually put the pounds back on again if they don't monitor their diet. Our brain develops a kind of memory of weight, which leads us to put on weight again once we stop dieting. In order to avoid putting the weight back on, here are some practical guidelines to follow:

- Remember that resuming normal eating habits does not mean you can slip back into excessive eating! Maintaining your weight means you promise yourself that you will not fall back to the same situation you were in before dieting.

- Continue to eat five low-calorie meals per week for the rest of your life. That's a small price to pay to stay slim!

- Monitor yourself regularly. Now that you've said adieu to your old clothes, your new wardrobe will help you to maintain your new waistline. If it becomes difficult to squeeze into your jeans or button a shirt, you'll know that you've gained weight.

- Weigh yourself once a week. If you've gained just a few extra pounds, get back on track with the recovery plan (see page 268). If you have gained more than four pounds above your Right Weight target, go back on the diet: use menus from the Café phase for two to three days (see pages 85–107), followed menus from the Bistro phase for a minimum of one week (see pages 109–163), and then menus from the Gourmet phase for a minimum of two weeks (see pages 165–257).

- Remember the basics of eating a balanced diet and the good habits you have acquired while dieting. Each time that you manage to avoid eating a high-calorie food and get just as much pleasure from a less rich one is a victory.

- Keep moving. Exercise is an ally in your fight against weight gain and looking fit. All forms of exercise are good: walking, running, going to the gym, swimming, cycling, the list is infinite. Thirty minutes of activity or more per day will keep you in shape. Give it everything you've got!

- Once you have successfully maintained your Right Weight for a minimum of six months to a year, you can set a new weight-loss goal by recalculating your Right Weight (taking into account your current stable weight) and start a new round of weight loss. This method of allowing your body to readjust over time will ensure that your weight-loss will be maintainable over the long term.

You will need to continue to monitor your weight in this way for the rest of your life. That may sound daunting, but just remember that you've chosen to be slim to please yourself. You haven't lost weight by chance, but because you had reasons for doing so and you worked hard at it. Making small changes now if you add on a little bit of weight is a lot easier than having to diet for an extended period of time every two or three years. You are in a good place. You have the power to stay here and continue to feel good about yourself. You've earned it.

Bon appétit!!

INDEX

ACKNOWLEDGMENTS

I would like to warmly thank:

My mother and father, who enabled me to pursue my education in the best possible conditions.

My wife Myriam and my three daughters, who have supported me through all of my "adventures" and whose love inspires me to surpass myself.

My editors, Kate Mascaro, Sophy Thompson, and Gilles Haéri, whose faith gives me courage and drive.

CharlElie Couture, who soothes me with his magnificent and inspiring music.

My American colleagues and friends, who honor me with their esteem.

My dear friends in New York: Jacob Sebag, Rachel Yohai, and the entire Larroche family, without forgetting Guy and Marie Dominique Sorman, who helped me understand that the U.S. truly is the country where anything is possible.

—Jean-Michel Cohen

The editor would like to thank Marnie Cochran for her invaluable advice, Meg Ragland for her judicious cuts, Thomas Gravemaker for his font research and constant support, nutritionist Barbara Rhys for her input, and the whole team whose contributions large and small made this book a reality.

THE PARISIAN DIET ONLINE

Calculate Your Right Weight with
Dr. Jean-Michel Cohen

To receive two weeks of free access to the Parisian Diet online weight-loss coaching program, go to **http://theparisiandiet.com/promo**

You will receive two weeks of free:
- coaching video sessions with Dr. Jean-Michel Cohen.
- personalized meal plans, recipes, and shopping lists.
- access to a vibrant and dynamic community of people just like you!

With Dr. Jean-Michel Cohen, Anxa.com has revolutionized the weight loss and fitness industry thanks to three key elements:
1. A proven nutritional diet based on clinical and scientific research.
2. A mobile app to motivate you to get involved for five minutes per day.
3. An online network that allows you to get to know yourself better, to interact with other users, and to carry out regular assessments related to your personal weight-loss goals.

To ensure that you get off to a great start, Anxa.com is pleased to offer you two weeks of free online support from Dr. Jean-Michel Cohen himself. Visit theparisiandiet.com/promo to start your free program right away. And if you have a Smartphone, download the application *The Parisian Diet* to your iPhone or Android phone.

Devour this fantastic book, adopt its tried-and-tested methods, and benefit from the online support with Dr. Jean-Michel Cohen and the team at Anxa.com.